Evaluation of N
Competence

Evaluation of
Nursing Competence

Harriet L. Schneider, R.N., M.Ed., Ed.D.

Associate Professor, Graduate Faculty, School of Nursing, University of Mississippi Medical Center, Jackson. Formerly Coordinator, Department of Test Development, National League for Nursing, New York

LITTLE, BROWN AND COMPANY, BOSTON

Library of Congress Catalog Card No. 78-73081

ISBN 0-316-77400-6

Printed in the United States of America

TO MY MOTHER WHO WOULD HAVE BEEN VERY PROUD

Preface

I suppose my interest in evaluation began when I was a nursing student and it was apparent to me that students were being graded not on their ability to give nursing care but on how the instructors felt about them. Similar situations seemed to occur in graduate school, too. The unfortunate part about that practice is that such evaluations tend to color those of others and may persist throughout the student's educational program—not to mention the effect such practices have on the individual! My own experiences as a head nurse, supervisor, and faculty member evaluating staff and students were fraught with dissatisfaction and questions about evaluation practices. Because of those occurrences as well as many comparable ones that I have been privy to in the course of conducting workshops and consulting with faculties on evaluation, I have written this book. It will, I hope, be helpful in remedying some of the gross injustices that take place in the name of evaluation.

Two very special people deserve my everlasting gratitude: Leonarda A. Laskevich (Lee) and M. Virginia Sellers (Ginny), friends and colleagues in the Department of Test Development, National League for Nursing, who helped in various ways to facilitate the completion of this book, including walking the dog. I am most appreciative of the interest and help of Marilyn A. Dees, also a consultant in the Department of Test Development, who assisted with the answers to the examination in Chapter 7. To Irving Robbins, friend, sounding board, and fan, my enduring thanks. To the faculty of the Downstate Medical Center College of Nursing in Brooklyn, New York, my sincere appreciation for involving me in the development of the videotape examination and then sharing the final results with me. Dr. Carla Mariano, a member of that faculty and later of the National League for Nursing Staff, provided the answers to the videotape examination. I have revised that test (in Chap. 5) in keeping with test construction principles.

I would be most interested in your comments, positive and negative, for those truly are in the realm of evaluation.

H. L. S.

Contents

Evaluation of Nursing Competence

1. Contributions to Assessment of Nursing Competence

Evaluating clinical competence in nursing is an old and perplexing problem. The need for instruments to measure competence is attested to in hundreds of articles as well as in many books, although the literature does contain a variety of approaches geared to resolving some of the problems involved. In addition to cost and time, the following problems are cited as being inherent in the evaluation of clinical performance: inconsistency between raters, low reliability of results obtained, defects in test validity, application of arbitrary standards, and weighting of some aspects of performance when such a procedure may not be warranted.

There have been a number of significant contributions, by individuals and groups, to the area of assessment of nursing performance, but none has provided complete solutions to the aforementioned problems. Before presenting examples of those contributions, however, the following definitions are offered so that the same baseline will be used by author and reader:

Competence "the quality or state of being functionally adequate or of having sufficient knowledge, judgment, skill, or strength [41, p. 463]."

Evaluation ". . . a process involving frequent use of different kinds of techniques . . . includes measurement but is broader in scope . . . an intellectual act [28]." Further, it is ". . . a systematic process of determining the extent to which educational objectives are achieved by pupils[14]."

Performance "the ability to perform: capacity to achieve a desired result: the act or process of carrying out something: the execution of an action [41]."

Urey [38] adapted a method of task analysis as a prelude to analyzing the entire range of nursing performance. Although a major undertaking, only six nursing procedures were analyzed. She stated that the following factors could or did alter performance: space, facilities, time, and stress.

Task analysis was also the method used by Dunn [7, p. 502] to develop rating checklists for five procedures. Each step in each checklist specifies the scientific principle involved. An additional feature is that each behavior is weighted according to its importance to the procedure, thus indicating that each step in a procedure may not be equally crucial. Evidence is presented relative to content validity and reliability, and, in particular, to inter-rater reliability. Two nurse-supervisors simultaneously and separately observed each nurse carrying out each procedure four times. High inter-rater reliability was obtained only when the observations were simultaneous. It is interesting to note that, due to cost and time factors, only 35 nurses were observed[7, p. 503].

A major study at the American Institutes for Research by Klaus and others [18] was geared toward improving nursing proficiency. The first report [18] established the rationale for the study, while a second identified 84 tasks, divided into 15 categories, that a general duty staff nurse working in a medical-surgical unit actually does [18]. A description of the performance of these tasks was to be used in evaluating nursing proficiency [19].

A third report [20] suggested a method for analyzing the tasks previously identified and described the various ways that nursing proficiency can be assessed. Only one task was analyzed, but the method utilized for the analysis is readily seen to be exhaustive and very time-consuming.

Another project emanating from the American Institutes for Research was directed and reported by Gorham [11, p. 68]. Flanagan's [9] critical incident technique was used as the basis for the design of the questionnaire. Almost 1,900 incidents were collected and subsequently classified into 15 categories of behavior in five major areas [11, p. 69]. The next step involved analyzing the incidents for behavioral components and then computing discrimination and affect values for the resulting 320 general behavioral statements. According to Gorham [12], the affect value was "an index of the degree to which each statement is a desirable behavior in relation to patient care." It was obtained by having a group of head nurses sort the statements into seven categories on a scale ranging from least to most descriptive of effective nursing performance [11, p. 75]. The discrimination value was "an index of the degree to which each statement empirically differentiates between the performance of the best nurses and that of the poorer nurses [12]." This was determined by asking head nurses to sort the statements into five categories indicating the degree to which each described the performance of a specified general staff nurse in her unit [11]. For the discrimination value, the reliability coefficient was reported to be .98 for the "good" nurse group and .90 for the "poor" group, with .97 for the affect value [11]. The followup report describes the six criterion instruments for measuring nursing performance developed on the basis of the earlier work, how the criterion instruments were administered and to whom, and, finally, the major findings of the study. Although the author states that the various procedures were "evaluated in terms of their relevance, reliability, rater 'errors,' objectivity, predictability, and acceptability," they are not reported [12].

Rines' [28] study, *Evaluating Student Progress in Learning the Practice of Nursing,* extended the theoretical base of evaluation by focusing on the why and how of such evaluation. Some 15 years after publication of her study, however, it appears that a considerable number of nurse-educators are still unfamiliar with the basic principles of evaluation. For example, Zasowska [44] studied the clinical laboratory experience in baccalaureate nursing programs and presented data on the evaluation of clinical performance. She found that since educational objectives were not used in planning clinical experiences, evaluation tended to be haphazard and irrelevant. There are, of course, many implications of such findings. An obvious one is that teachers of nursing need to be prepared for their evaluation responsibilities.

Further validation of Zasowska's findings are presented in a study of the laboratory concept in baccalaureate nursing programs by Infante [17], who reported that only 53 percent of faculty responding to her questionnaire said that they had specific objectives for clinical laboratory experience. It is interesting to note that of the 53 percent, about less than half apprised students of those objectives.

A project to improve evaluation and prediction of clinical performance was undertaken in a diploma nursing program. Heins and her faculty [15, p. 117], with the assistance of a consultant group, developed 12 rating scales and two global instruments ". . . to assist in validating the specialized clinical instruments. These instruments were the Effective-Ineffective Scale and the Role Nomination form." The clinical rating was on a 0-to-5 scale and provided anchoring descriptions of each value [15, p. 18]. Although a large amount of data was presented relative to reliability and validity, the majority dealt with the intercorrelations of rating scales (either the entire scale or total scale subcategories). Although scale revisions were done on the basis of early data, subsequent reliability measurements involved only small numbers of students. However, some of the behaviors were not really appropriate on a form to evaluate nursing performance by direct observation; many could be better evaluated by means of paper-and-pencil tests in the less expensive environment of the classroom. Despite this, the positive results from this project would be helpful to other groups coping with a comparable problem.

Gerchberg [10] undertook a small-scale project to improve evaluation of her nursing students. She describes four methods used to assist students with self-evaluation as well as to improve data collection by their teachers. The behavioral observations involve direct observation by the teacher, assignment of a nursing care plan, the keeping of a nursing diary, and a nursing process recording by the student. A detailed account is given of the evaluation method employed with 2 of the 10 students involved in the project and relates the objectives for clinical laboratory experiences to the method used. Although no solution is given to any of the problems of performance evaluation (most projects on performance evaluation do not provide any), and bearing in mind that the study was limited to 10 students in one diploma school of nursing, the approach still was basically sound as well as commendable in its attempt.

A numerical rating scale to measure nurse competency was constructed by Slater [31]. It consists of 84 items separated into six categories and can be used either retrospectively for varying periods of time or for a two and one-half hour period as a nurse provides on-the-spot patient care. The specificity of the behaviorally defined items is one stated means of making the scale more objective. The manual that accompanies the scale reports a split-half reliability of .985 and states that further testing of inter-rater reliability will be done. Failure of this long and complex tool to be universally accepted appears to be related to the fact that evaluation by direct observation is time-consuming, a common criticism of such evaluative devices. (See the published version [40] .)

The same criticism is also applicable to Dyer's tool for evaluating nursing performance [8] . The Nurse Performance Description Scales contains 50 items in 16 categories, each category on a dimension of nursing care, and consists of descriptive statements of typical behavior along a continuum. Each nurse to be evaluated is given a score of from 1 to 11, with all nurses to be evaluated on one category before proceeding to the next. Designed for research purposes over an eight-year period, the tool was subjected to checks of its reliability and validity. Test-retest reliability ranged from .80 to .88 in the four sample hospitals, and three checks of concurrent validity are presented in the report [8, p. 215].

Tate and her colleagues [34, 35] worked for three to four years on an evaluation form that later was subjected to validity and reliability studies. In spite of reports of high reliability (the lowest scale reliability was .972), "excellent discrimination [35, p. 75] ," and at least two explanatory articles in nursing journals [32, 33] , the form has not been widely accepted and, to my knowledge, now lies essentially dormant.

A recently ended project funded by the United States Office of Education at the University of California at Los Angeles developed instructional materials for the allied health professions, including the associate degree nursing student [42, p. 11] . One aspect of the project included the development of tests of performance and performance checklists, the latter designed for use in the learning laboratory and later in the clinical setting. The project staff broke down the nursing curriculum into three levels: "Level I—entry-level nursing skills; Level II—comparable to present LVN (LPN) curricula; Level III—comparable to present registered nurse curricula [42, p. 6] ." The progress report included a sample of a performance test for "Handwashing Technique for Medical Asepsis [42, p. 73] ," which stated *only* the following: "In the skill laboratory you will correctly demonstrate the handwashing procedure, carefully observing the proper sequence of steps listed in the procedure [42, p. 73] ." Also included is a performance checklist for the same procedure [42, pp. 54, 74] . It will be interesting to read followup reports of this project because materials were being developed for all levels of nurses through those having or holding doctorates. As of mid 1978, however, no further reports have been released on the various levels of nurses. Books have been published that are procedurally oriented, helpful to the nursing profession in and of themselves [43] . Those procedures are useful both for learning and for designing an evaluation tool to assess competency in carrying out those procedures.

Simpson [30] describes a "walk around" practical examination for evaluating basic clinical nursing skills. Patients are not used. Equipment is displayed, and students are told by cards next to each setup what information they are to record on their answer sheets. Although this method seems appropriate for determining if students can read a thermometer, in order to assess more complex skills situations would need to be structured in such a way that students would be able to demonstrate the desired behaviors.

A search of the literature revealed several studies—conducted in various fields, although only one pertaining to nursing—that employ a movie test of some type. Although each had its own purpose, the findings, as interpreted by me, suggest potential application to nursing. These research findings on simulation coupled with some from the fields of medicine, education, management, economics, politics, and the military would indicate that simulation techniques for evaluating clinical nursing competence are both possible and desirable. Such assessment tools could provide nursing educators with information about the clinical competence of students and staff not now possible to obtain.

The only study that did pertain specifically to nursing, reported in *Nursing Outlook* [21], utilizes a teaching film as the basis for an essay examination on patient-care problems. Nursing students used the film *The Special Universe of Walter Krolik* (cosponsored by the National Tuberculosis Association, the American Nurses' Association, and the National League for Nursing) to identify problems from cues given by the patient. This standardized patient situation was used to evaluate the student's ability to perform one facet of the nursing process, the assessment phase. Following the identification of the cues and problems, students designed a nursing care plan, listing both the action to be taken and its rationale.

In her study, Davis [4] employed a 16-mm film consisting of five segments (each of them one or two minutes long) in which different patient situations were shown. The object was to have registered nurses with different educational preparation record the observations they made, the action they would take, and the reason for those actions. The film had been developed earlier by Verhonick and others [39] to assess the responses of nurses to filmed patient situations; their study also related the nurse's level of education to the frequency of relevant observations. Davis' [4] hypothesis—that the quantity and quality of patient care provided by clinical nurse specialists would be superior to that provided by baccalaureate nurses—was supported. Davis replicated this study in 1974 obtaining similar results [5].

Other studies have described the development of simulated clinical nursing tests for assessing the problem-solving skills of the nurse, although these have been confined to written descriptions of the situation. For example, McIntyre and associates [25] designed an 81-item test in two parts, one a controlled-response and the other a free-response section. The entire test was based on the needs of one patient over a period of time. Five scoring systems were developed, each for a different purpose. Scoring Systems I and II assessed the quality of clinical judgment [25]. While they agree that clinical evaluation is in need of strengthening, their test gets at knowledge, not performance.

Of course the nursing profession has not been alone in its concern with and striving for an improvement in performance evaluation. The professions of medicine and teaching too have been undergoing critical reviews of their prevailing assessment measures. Popham [26, 27] has been especially critical of the techniques used to evaluate the performance of teachers. He has, however, taken giant strides in devising measures to overcome those shortcomings and also to publicize both the existing deficiencies and some ways to remedy them [26]. The major theme of his work has been use of a performance-based evaluation or an "outcomes-focused approach" [27] as opposed to "more process-focused strategies [27]." Unfortunately, teaching performance tests have not been recommended for the evaluation of individual teachers but rather are more useful for assessing the efficacy of teacher education programs. As Popham himself has stated [27, p. 71] the key elements of what constitutes competent teaching are yet to be delineated.

Medical educators, recognizing the necessity of measuring clinical competence, have developed a variety of tests, among them the Programmed (sequential) Test and a test that employed motion pictures of selected patients. These two tests were developed by the National Board of Medical Examiners and constituted Part III of their examination for some time [16]. The motion picture test purported to control one variable (the patient) by projecting him on a screen and to control the other variable (the bedside examiner) by the provision of pretested multiple-choice questions. One stated advantage is that such films simulate the real-life situation.

Levine and McGuire [22] have developed a simulation examination for physicians that employs role-playing techniques. They claim that: (1) such an examination has the face validity of a patient interview, (2) simulation assures that all examinees are presented with the same clinical problem, and (3) performance standards can be established. Since such a technique involved a two-day training period for the examiner and since one of the methods used yielded an unreliable rating (the other two were .58 and .72), it would appear that further refinement is indicated.

Another simulation technique devised by McGuire and Babbott [24, p. 1] involves the measurement of problem-solving skills and is "designed to measure aspects of behavior defined by a criterion group as essential components of clinical competence." Reliabilities range from .75 to .94 depending on the length of the test(s). Preliminary results from the validity studies suggest that this technique is of value for its stated purpose [24, p. 9].

Barrows [1] has devised an interesting technique for assessing the competence of neurologists. He has "programmed" actors to simulate patients with neurological problems. One of the advantages of this approach is that medical students and doctors are now able to see clinical problems not otherwise available because of their rarity or, if available, detrimental to the patient (e.g., a grand mal seizure may be triggered in a patient as a result of the stress associated with being observed by a group of doctors and students); another advantage is that information about a physician's skills never before observable can now be obtained.

A trained observer is necessary, although he does not have to be a physician. Reports are obtained from both the observer and the "patient," and a final evaluation by the physician's instructor is arrived at on the basis of these two reports. Some of the problems of other observational techniques such as time and subjectivity also apply to this technique however.

Some 30 years ago Thorndike [36] discussed the merits of motion pictures for presenting test material, specifying among them their realism when compared with printed information. He also cited the extensive exploration of this area by the Aviation Psychology Program of the Army Air Force. Studies in which motion pictures are the basis for subsequent test questions have existed for a number of years, but only within the last 10 to 15 years have films become sophisticated enough for any purpose other than supplemental teaching. For example, Seibert and colleagues [29] described "an analysis of film's contribution to the factor analytic study of human intellect." They used 49 films of various cinematographic techniques, including animation, and of various durations, some only milliseconds long, to test their hypotheses on visual memory, serial cognition, and operation hierarchies. One fairly consistent finding in studies such as this is that films effectively impart information dealing with action and activity [2]. Another idea that permeates the literature on media application is that films may be able to measure objectives that static stimuli cannot [23].

Psychometricians and organizations concerned with testing, for example, the Educational Testing Service, have developed measurement instruments to minimize the subjective and time-consuming elements associated with observation scales. Improvement has been achieved by the provision of guides and by rather extensive training of the persons who will do the observing, but the reliability of these scales is still seriously low.

The remaining chapters examine a variety of methods of obtaining information about the knowledge base of nurses. Since one of the maxims of evaluation is to gather as much valid information as possible in order to obtain a reliable measure of competence, many tools may need to be employed in arriving at a decision about an individual's competence. Bear in mind that the examples that follow may serve only as models in many instances and will need to be modified or adapted to the requirements of the individual school or institution. Subject matter, curriculum organization or design, institutional policies, the philosophy of the faculty, and the like will all affect the ultimate design and product and rightly so. No tool is likely to be universally accepted in toto and should not be expected to be *the* ultimate one.

REFERENCES

1. Barrows, H. S. *Simulated Patients (Programmed Patients): The Development and Use of a New Technique in Medical Education.* Springfield, Ill.: Charles C Thomas, 1971.
2. Briggs, L., Campeau, P., Gagne, R., and May, M. *Instructional Media: A Procedure for the Design of Multi-Media Instruction, A Critical*

Review of Research, and Suggestions for Future Research. Pittsburgh: American Institutes for Research, 1967. P. 115.

3. Cronbach, L. J.   *Essentials of Psychological Testing* (3rd ed.). New York: Harper & Row, 1970. P. 27.

4. Davis, B. G.   Clinical expertise as a function of educational preparation. *Nurs. Res.* 21:530, 1972.

5. Davis, B. G.   Effect of levels of nursing education on patient care: A replication. *Nurs. Res.* 23:150–155, 1974.

6. deTornyay, R.   Measuring problem-solving skills by means of the simulated clinical nursing problem test. *J. Nurs. Educ.* 7:3, 1968.

7. Dunn, M.   Development of an instrument to measure nursing performance. *Nurs. Res.* 19:502–503, 1970.

8. Dyer, E. D.   Nurse Performance Description: Criteria, Predictors, and Correlates. In *Fifth Nursing Research Conference.* Proceedings of the Fifth Nursing Research Conference, New Orleans, La., March 3–5, 1969. Pp. 208–233.

9. Flanagan, J. C.   The critical incident technique. *Psychol. Bull.* 51:327, 1954.

10. Gerchberg, L. R.   *An Observational Method for Evaluating the Performance of Nursing Students in Clinical Situations* (League Exchange No. 60). New York: National League for Nursing, 1962.

11. Gorham, W. A.   Staff nursing behaviors contributing to patient care and improvement. *Nurs. Res.* 11:68–69, 75, 1962.

12. Gorham, W. A.   Methods for measuring staff nursing performance. *Nurs. Res.* 12:4, 1963.

13. Gover, V. F.   The Development and Testing of a Nursing Performance Simulation Instrument. Ed.D. dissertation, University of North Carolina at Chapel Hill, 1971.

14. Gronlund, N. E.   *Measurement and Evaluation in Teaching* (2nd ed.). New York: Macmillan, 1971. P. 8.

15. Heins, M. J., Hawk, T., Busch, J., DeRidder, L., Flitter, H., and Ray, J. *Evaluation and Prediction of Clinical Performance in a School of Nursing.* Knoxville, Tenn.: St. Mary's Memorial Hospital School of Nursing, 1971. Pp. 18, 117.

16. Hubbard, J.   Programmed Testing in the Examinations of the National Board of Medical Examiners. In *Proceedings of the 1963 Invitational Conference on Testing Problems.* Princeton, N.J.: Educational Testing Service, 1964. Pp. 52–53.

17. Infante, M. S.   The Laboratory Concept in Baccalaureate Education in Nursing. Ed.D. dissertation, Teachers College, Columbia University, 1972. P. 102.

18. Klaus, D. J., Gosnell, D. E., Jacobs, A. M., Reilly, P. C., and Taylor, J. A.   *Controlling Experience to Improve Nursing Proficiency: Background and Study Plans.* Report No. 1. Pittsburgh: American Institutes for Research, 1966.

19. Klaus, D. J., Gosnell, D. E., Reilly, P. C., and Taylor, J. A.   *Controlling Experience to Improve Nursing Proficiency: Categories of Nursing Performance.* Report No. 2. Pittsburgh: American Institutes for Research, 1968.

20. Klaus, D. J., Gosnell, D. E., Reilly, P. C., and Chowla, M. J.   *Controlling Experience to Improve Nursing Proficiency: Determining Proficient Performance.* Report No. 3. Pittsburgh: American Institutes for Research, 1968.

21. Kubo, W., Chase, L., and Leton, J.   A creative examination. *Nurs. Outlook* 19:524, 1971.

22. Levine, H. G., and McGuire, C. H.   Role-playing as an evaluative technique. *J. Educ. Measure* 5:1, 1968.
23. Loughary, J.   *Man-Made Systems in Education.* New York: Harper & Row, 1966. P. 75.
24. McGuire, C. H., and Babbott, D.   Simulation techniques in the measurement of problem-solving skills. *J. Educ. Measure* 4:1, 9, 1967.
25. McIntyre, H., McDonald, F., Bailey, J., and Claus, K.   A simulated clinical nursing test. *Nurs. Res.* 21:429, 1972.
26. Popham, W. J.   Performance tests of teaching proficiency: Rationale, development, and validation. *Am. Educ. Res. J.* 8:105, 1971.
27. Popham, W. J.   Minimal competencies for objectives-oriented teacher education programs. *J. Teach. Educ.* 25:68, 71, 1974.
28. Rines, A. R.   *Evaluating Student Progress in Learning the Practice of Nursing.* New York: Teachers College Press, 1963. Pp. 8–9.
29. Seibert, W. F., Snow, R. E., and Senn, J. L., Jr.   *Studies in Cine-Psychometry 1:Preliminary Factor Analysis of Visual Cognition and Memory.* Lafayette, Ind.: Purdue University Audio-Visual Center, 1965. P. 2.
30. Simpson, M. J.   The walk-around laboratory practical examination in evaluating clinical nursing skills. *J. Nurs. Educ.* 6:23, 1967.
31. Slater, D.   *The Slater Nursing Competencies Rating Scale.* Detroit: Wayne State University College of Nursing, 1967. P. 12.
32. Tate, B. L.   Evaluating the nurse's clinical performance. *Nurs. Outlook* 10:35, 1962.
33. Tate, B. L.   Evaluation of clinical performance of the staff nurse. *Nurs. Res.* 11:7, 1962.
34. Tate, B. L.   *A Method for Rating the Proficiency of the Hospital General Staff Nurse.* New York: National League for Nursing, 1964.
35. Tate, B. L.   *Test of a Nursing Performance Evaluation Instrument.* New York: National League for Nursing, 1964. P. 75.
36. Thorndike, R. L.   *Personnel Selection.* New York: Wiley & Sons, 1949. P. 42.
37. Thorndike, R. L., and Hagen, E.   *Measurement and Evaluation in Psychology and Education* (4th ed.). New York: Wiley & Sons, 1977.
38. Urey, B. I.   A Method for Analysis of Nursing Tasks. Ed.D. dissertation, Teachers College, Columbia University, 1968. Pp. 116–120.
39. Verhonick, P., Nichols, G., Glor, B., and McCarthy, R.   I came, I saw, I responded: Nursing observation and action survey. *Nurs. Res.* 17:38, 1968.
40. Wandelt, M. A., and Slater Stewart, D.   *Slater Nursing Competencies Rating Scale.* New York: Appleton-Century-Crofts, 1975.
41. *Webster's Third New International Dictionary of the English Language, Unabridged.* Springfield, Mass.: G. & C. Merriam, 1964. Pp. 463, 1678, 2122.
42. Wood, L. A., and Freeland, T. E.   *The UCLA Allied Health Professions Projects: Nursing Occupations Progress Report.* Los Angeles: University of California, 1971. Pp. 6, 11, 54, 73–74.
43. Wood, L. A., and Rambo, B. J. (Eds.).   *Nursing Skills for Allied Health Services* (2nd ed.). Philadelphia: W. B. Saunders, 1977.
44. Zasowska, M. A.   A Descriptive Survey of Significant Factors in the Clinical Laboratory Experience in Baccalaureate Education for Nursing. Ed.D. dissertation, Teachers College, Columbia University, 1967. Pp. 188–199.

2. Evaluation of Clinical Competence in Nursing

When discussing the evaluation of clinical competence in nursing, an apt direction to take can be found in the title of Merwin's presidential address to the National Council of Measurement in Education in 1972, "Educational Measurement of What Characteristic of Whom (or What) by Whom and Why [3]." To complete the picture for its use in nursing, other facets will be added, namely "when," "how," and "where." Only selected aspects of each will be considered, however.

Whenever clinical competence is to be assessed, certain assumptions must be made:

1. Evaluation of clinical competence by direct observation in the clinical laboratory presupposes that the nursing student has had the opportunity to learn before he or she is evaluated on performance.
2. Competence in the actual clinical situation presupposes sufficient knowledge to take appropriate action.
3. The total milieu of the real-life clinical setting cannot be replicated in a simulated situation.
4. Paper-and-pencil tests can only measure the cognitive aspects of the total constellation of behavior inherent in the practice of nursing.
5. The answers selected by the examinee in a paper-and-pencil test reflect only what he chose in that particular instance and cannot be interpreted to mean that he would actually take the chosen action in a real-life situation.

These assumptions will be discussed in more detail as the chapter progresses.

WHY EVALUATE?

Before any action to evaluate is taken, the primary questions to be answered are the "of whom" and "why," since they are intertwined. For example, the purpose behind evaluating a general-duty staff nurse, with the why being to determine whether a salary increase is deserved, is quite different from that behind evaluating a nursing student to determine if he or she has mastered the principles of medical asepsis. Cronbach [2] and others say, in reference to the why, evaluation is done chiefly to assess the attainment of unit, course, and program objectives. It entails both formative and summative evaluation. Although Bloom and his associates [1] have devoted an entire book to the subject, a brief and gross distinction between the two types of evaluation is that formative evaluation denotes "diagnostic-progress tests and summative evaluation achievement examinations." It is unfortunate that in practice the emphasis has been on summative evaluation, that is, the kind done at the end of a course, usually too late for the instructor to remedy problems that require remedial attention. Focusing more than has generally been done on the formative aspects of evaluation (done as the student is progressing) would enable instructors to make evaluation more like what it should be, constructive.

In addition to affirming that nursing students are ready to progress to the next level in the school program, evaluation allows faculty to state with a degree of confidence that graduates of their program are competent nursing practitioners and are ready to sit for the State Board Test Pool Examination, one of the requisites for obtaining a license to practice as a registered nurse. This latter step, evaluation by faculty prior to graduation, is an essential one, since the licensing examination is a paper-and-pencil test that measures only a minimum level of safety and effectiveness of nursing practice. It also covers only a sample of the universe of nursing content. It measures only what the nurse knows, not what he or she does (or will do). Therefore, graduation from a school of nursing should be synonymous with demonstrated nursing competence—cognitive *and* behavioral.

Underlying the why of summative evaluation, then, is the need to guarantee the recipients of nursing care competence in that care. This is particularly relevant at this time because of the numerous discussions and proposals relative to relicensure of nurses.

THE PROCESS OF EVALUATION

The next question to be answered is the "what" of evaluation. Almost every nursing program includes nonnursing as well as nursing content, but this what will be concerned with nursing content only.* The two major requisites for clinical competence in nursing are knowledge and the ability to perform, neither of which is mutually exclusive. The constellation of behaviors necessary for nursing includes not only knowledge and psycho-motor abilities, but also attitudes and cognitive skills such as problem-solving. Assessment should encompass essential aspects from among the repertoire of behaviors; obviously those behaviors need to be observable in order to be measured. It is important to sample all categories of behavior, since, for example, the nurse who *knows* how to suction a tracheostomy may not be able to *do* it (assuming that the nurse has the necessary manual dexterity, that he or she is physically able to carry out the procedure, and that circumstances do not thwart his or her performance). A nurse who knows that women in labor are apprehensive but does nothing to allay that apprehension is clinically incompetent, unable to apply what he or she "knows."

Knowing what to evaluate—knowledge and performance—leads to the problem of *how* to evaluate those abilities. Although there are many evaluation methods, including oral examinations and patient-care studies (the

*Many nursing programs purport to incorporate knowledge from other disciplines into the nursing courses, and the degree to which that is done would obviously need to be taken into account in any assessment.

latter an effective approach for assessing the cognitive level of synthesis), discussion will be limited to paper-and-pencil and performance tests.

Paper-and-pencil tests can accurately measure what the nurse knows, assuming that the rules of test construction are used in designing the test. These rules include representativeness of the sample from the universe of content, making process levels more demanding than the trivial recall of facts and minutiae, and unambiguously stating test questions. Both teacher-made and national, standardized tests have their place in the evaluation of nursing knowledge. Both can be very sophisticated, psychometrically sound instruments and can provide valuable information on what a student or group of students know. While the teacher-made tests obviously emphasize content the instructor deems important and to which she is committed, the standardized ones enable the instructor, among other things, to compare what she feels is important to that deemed important by a great number of other instructors throughout the country in comparable educational programs.

One real advantage of the standardized test is that it is well constructed when compared to the average teacher-made test and is therefore likely to more accurately measure whatever it is measuring. With a teacher-made test the test-wise student can often figure out what the teacher wants for an answer or can determine the correct answer by eliminating each of the distracters (wrong options). If the same teacher-made examinations are used year after year, the practice in some schools, there is the problem of the dissemination of content from class to class so that attained scores are not true measures of students' knowledge.

On the other hand, evaluating what the nurse can *do* is beset with difficulties. Assuming that instruments designed to measure behavior are well constructed and that work samples are adequate and representative, there is still one big problem, namely, the necessity of direct observation of the performance. The observation time required to sample the behaviors of a nurse is extensive, and when one multiplies the time required by the number of students in the class or staff on the clinical unit, it is no wonder that some instructors and supervisors balk at the task. The time factor plus the lack of appropriate tools result in clinical performance evaluations that are often subjective, vague, unreliable, inappropriate, and ineffective.

Part of the problem of ineffective performance evaluation is due to the fact that many aspects of performance are evaluated in the clinical laboratory when they could be more efficiently evaluated in the college learning laboratory. This, then, gets to the point of "where" to evaluate. There would seem to be no problem with where to test cognition: in the college classroom. Rather, the major problem appears to be the inappropriate use of the clinical laboratory for evaluating all types of performance. The ability to perform basic psychomotor skills coupled with the related cognitive components of those skills is best accomplished in the college learning laboratory. A very simple example is assessing the ability of a student to take a patient's temperature and to read the thermometer accurately. It is a poor use of the clinical laboratory experience to evaluate this ability there unless there are other objectives involved. If more evaluation were done in the college learning laboratory when it is appropriate to do so, the information gathered when evaluating students' performances in the clinical laboratory would be more meaningful than it now generally is. Significant time per student would also be saved if observation were confined to only what should be evaluated in that situation.

As is true in the construction of a test question, specificity is essential in the design of a tool to measure performance. Some faculty members and supervising nurses believe that if performance is broken down into its component parts, it is something less than professional, in fact unprofessional. But how does one determine if a nurse "uses the nursing process in the care of patients" unless each of the steps involved in the nursing process is listed and defined to the extent that it can be said unequivocally that a nurse either does or does not take a specific action?

The next question to be answered pertains more to evaluation of clinical performance than to assessing cognitive competence and is relatively easy to answer. In the case of nursing students, the "by whom" in the majority of instances should be the faculty responsible for course content. It has been the practice in some schools to hire an adjunct faculty member to evaluate certain aspects of performance in the laboratory, one advantage of which is to free the master teacher for other scholarly pursuits. On the other hand, such an observer is not likely to be familiar with what students have been taught. In many such circumstances there has been no continuity from classroom to clinical laboratory, thus putting the student in an awkward position.

Another point to be considered is that educationally and philosophically it is not sound practice to have head nurses and supervisors evaluate the clinical performance of students unless the nurses and supervisors have been temporarily freed of their administrative responsibilities for the time necessary to do the evaluation. There may otherwise be a conflict of objectives—education versus service (patient care).

The question of "when" to evaluate may not seem to be as crucial as some of the other questions, but it does need to be mentioned. A maxim of evaluation—applicable to both cognitive and performance evaluation—not universally adhered to is that it should take place only after the student has had the opportunity to learn. In addition, short tests—paper-and-pencil or performance—on just one segment of the course aid both student and instructor in assessing both trouble spots in need of remediation as well as those areas relatively problem-free. Such tests are likely to reduce the number of students who fail course-end examinations, always assuming that corrective measures had been taken during the course and that the final examination is both reliable and valid for the intended purpose.

The when of nursing staff performance evaluation may well be determined by institutional policy. A common practice is having an evaluation after a probationary period of, say, three months, another in six months, and yearly thereafter. Staff should be apprised of the prevailing policy when first employed and should receive, well before the evaluation is to be done, both the actual form that will be used and the guidelines that accompany the evaluation form. This practice is intended to make the process of evaluation less frustrating and fraught with anxiety for both the evaluator and the person being assessed and to place evaluation in a positive light rather than in its all too often negative position.

Other Ways of Evaluating Competence

Because of the many problems inherent in clinical performance evaluation and because of the many advantages of paper-and-pencil testing, we should try to utilize those advantages of objective testing. One way would be to combine a paper-and-pencil test with a simulated clinical setting. A paper-and-pencil test based on the content of a simulated clinical situation including some of the course objectives not testable by conventional paper-and-pencil tests would cut back on the time involved in direct observation of a student's performance.

A simulation could present the students with a situation they have not encountered before, thus testing application of gained knowledge. When answering questions based on that stimulus, the nursing student would be responding much as he or she would in the actual clinical situation. The cues presented by a patient in a real situation require a response, sometimes without clarification of the cues. A sound film presenting a patient situation would require students to respond to actual behavior rather than to a *description* of behavior, which, in the case of a paper-and-pencil test, is behavior in the abstract. The test could include questions on the adequacy of the performance of the nurses in the film, the appropriateness of the nurses' responses to the patient, and alternate methods of achieving patient-care goals.

Theoretically, then, the student or nurse who scored high on a simulation test could be expected to demonstrate a higher level of competence in that clinical area than the student or nurse who scored low. The basis for this theory is that a student or nurse who is likely to provide nursing care in an acceptable manner herself would be more likely to recognize acceptable nursing behavior in a film. Conversely, if a student or nurse would be more apt to behave incompetently, she would be less likely to recognize incompetent behavior. Other advantages of such standardized simulation tests are that (1) each student or nurse can respond to the same situation, and (2) there would be less involvement with semantics and less ambiguity in the interpretation as compared to the written description.

The following specifications and characteristics should all be considered when developing a standardized simulation test:

1. It should be appropriate for mass administration.
2. Short-answer objective test items should be used.
3. Administration can be accomplished in a short time, for example, during a class period.
4. Scoring can be done by machine or easily by hand, and quantification of the results is possible.
5. Faculty interpretation of the results is relatively easy.

6. Reliability is comparable to that of other standardized nursing tests.
7. Validity for assessing clinical competence in the area specified approaches or surpasses that of other standardized nursing tests.

A more detailed discussion of testing based on films as well as the use of existing films for such tests and the production of "test" films is presented in Chapter 3. A test of this type based on a clinical labor and delivery situation is also given.

REFERENCES
1. Bloom, B. S., Hastings, J. H., and Madaus, G. F. *Handbook on Formative and Summative Evaluation of Student Learning.* New York: McGraw-Hill, 1971. P. 56.
2. Cronbach, L. J. Course improvement through evaluation. *Teach. Coll. Rec.* 64:672, 1963.
3. Merwin, J. C. Education measurement of what characteristic of whom (or what) by whom and why. *J. Educ. Measure.* 10:1, 1973.

3. Tests Based on Films

Using films in a test or instructional situation is not a new idea. Some 30 years ago Robert Thorndike [22] wrote of the advantages of presenting a stimulus or situation in a motion picture and stated that the realism was superior to that of the written word. Seibert, Snow, and Senn [20] in 1965 reported on the use of films to test various facets of human intellect, including memory and cognition. Others, such as Briggs and colleagues [6] in 1967, used films in a variety of instructional methods and conducted research on their use. They concluded that films are very effective in presenting information related to action.

The advantages of films are many but perhaps the most important one is that they depict real situations that can be shown to an audience when the same live situation is not available. Perhaps the best example of this is the birth of a baby—women do not always have babies when nursing students are scheduled to have their labor and delivery experience. Another advantage is that films can compress time. Although a woman's labor may last many hours, the filmed sequence of that labor can be shortened to minutes but still be effectively portrayed. In comparison with other visual media, the quality and clarity of film is usually superior, particularly when projected on a large screen. There is better definition in the movie print than in a videotape, for example. If the film is to be used for purposes of observation and subsequent testing, it is necessary for the film to be of the highest quality possible because any defects will interfere with those observations and will thereby obfuscate the intended purpose. For example, an inexperienced cameraman is more likely to build in inadvertently factors such as jerking camera movements that will interfere with subsequent viewing. Another advantage of films is that they are relatively indestructible, in fact, extremely durable. No special considerations other than adequate storage facilities are necessary.

Probably the biggest disadvantage of making one's own films is the cost of production, a recent cost estimate being $1,400 per minute. If then one were interested in making a 15-minute color film, the proposed cost of $21,000 could well change one's mind. Part of this high cost is due to the need to shoot many more feet of film than will actually be used in the final product. With film one has to wait until the film is developed to see the results, as opposed to the immediate feedback of videotape, so it is less expensive to shoot extra footage initially than to reconstruct the situation.

Another disadvantage is that films need to be shown in relative darkness, making note-taking difficult, if not impossible. The sound (audio) portion of films may be a problem, and thus a disadvantage, particularly in the single-concept type and in homemade movies. If the audio portion is transcribed to the optical track after the film is developed, the sound may be "out of sync," i.e., not synchronized with lip movements, although this problem is not as likely to occur in professionally produced films. If such distortion is marked, verbal cues and body cues would be in conflict, thus causing possible confusion to the observer. If magnetic audiotape is transferred to the optical track, thus minimizing the chance of this happening, an additional expense is incurred.

If after weighing the advantages and disadvantages of films, it is decided to use a film for the purpose of testing, the next decision to be made is whether to make one (either by yourself or with a professional producer) or to use what is already available.

MAKING YOUR OWN FILM

If the decision is to make a film, a script must be written. A decided advantage of making one's own film is that its specifications can be defined to meet your needs, thereby controlling the film's content. If the aim of the film is to depict a clinical situation, one can put into the script examples of both competent and incompetent nursing performance. Either accurate or inaccurate, or both, subject matter can also be included, again to meet the objectives. Although both extremes of the continuum have been cited, there is no limit to what can be included along that continuum. Much depends upon what one wishes to test. Since the purpose of the film will be to test knowledge needed by nurses, there should be no irrelevant and extraneous material (a common finding in existing films). In writing the script, one must keep in mind the purpose of the film; for example, if a real-life situation is to be faithfully simulated, some of the typical sounds and sights of a hospital unit should probably be included.

Depending upon what and how much one wishes to test, it may be possible to write a script that will cover the desired content completely yet concisely, with the resulting film still being relatively short, a decided advantage. After a lengthy film, observers may be hard put to remember all that has occurred in it. Several short but complete films are probably better for purposes of testing than one long one.

As with any test, content validation is essential and so it would be desirable to have the script content validated. If a group of nursing experts in a particular area has been involved in defining the content for the script and has contributed to its evaluation, there has been a built-in process of content validation. On the other hand, if the script has been written by only one faculty member, it is wise indeed to have one or more (preferably more) experts on that subject validate the content. Such a process will be less expensive in the long run since some of the "bugs" will be taken care of *before* filming.

Once the script has been approved, shooting of the film can begin. One would assume that a commercial producer has already been engaged, if one is to be used. Using professionally competent actors adds to the realism of the film. It also avoids the problem of having the audience laugh at the poor acting ability of some inexperienced or frightened novices, thus distracting viewers from the content of the film. The entire process of making the film will be facilitated by such professional assistance. If, however, the film is to be made by nursing faculty, help may be available from the audiovisual center of the college, knowledgeable faculty outside of nursing, or friends and acquaintances not within the university setting. Many recent books on the subject of film-making are a valuable source of information and guidance. Some such publications are listed at the end of this chapter.

SELECTION AND USE OF AN EXISTING FILM

Before one starts the search for a film, a task more difficult than would appear, criteria of what is wanted in a film should be established. For example, the following criteria were used when I was looking for a film around which I ultimately developed the test for assessing baccalaureate students in nursing programs over a geographically dispersed sample.

1. The situation depicted must parallel one likely to be encountered by most baccalaureate nursing students in the course of their education.
2. Nurses should be seen performing the kinds of activities customarily expected in that situation.
3. The dialogues between nurse and patient and nurse and physician must be extensive enough to permit judgments to be made.
4. Content from a variety of disciplines (albeit all related to the situation) would be desirable; for example, sociological, psychological, and physiological subject matter were felt to be necessary.
5. The content did not have to be medically accurate nor the performance of nurses without flaw, since questions could be directed toward any inadequacies.
6. The subject matter contained in the film should be either in the field of pediatric nursing or in obstetric nursing because of my experience in these fields.
7. The quality of the film's sound and photography must be such that the "surround" (noise and other extraneous subject matter) would not interfere with an examinee's performance on the test.

The next step was to review 152 film synopses that had been compiled in conjunction with teaching courses in Maternal and Child Nursing over a 14-year period. Only one film seemed to be suitable for the project, but it was eliminated upon being re-viewed.

The National Survey of Audiovisual Materials for Nursing [19] of 1970 was then consulted. Among the 10 16-mm films listed for pediatric nursing, several were on growth and development and several on maternal deprivation; of the remaining ones, none involved a nurse actually taking care of a child. In the obstetric nursing section there were 11 16-mm films listed, including films on emergency deliveries, breast-feeding, the problems of an Rh negative-sensitized woman, and a 20-year-old film on nurse-midwifery. Only one involved nursing care and this one was finally selected as the stimulus for the test to be developed.* The 30-minute film, *Birth Day—Through the Eyes of the Mother* [3], portrays a woman admitted to the hospital in early labor and follows her through the delivery of her infant. It is a 16-mm, commercially made color and sound motion picture. The technique used in making the film, subjective camera or cinema verite (through the eyes of the beholder), depicts a real patient in the process of having a baby. The film accurately reflects the kind of situation likely to occur in most hospitals with labor and delivery facilities.

In addition to the criteria previously cited, it was felt that what was covered in the film—a normal labor and delivery—was appropriate as the basis for a test because the objectives of courses in obstetric nursing are fairly consistent in most baccalaureate programs, regardless of the title of the course. Such a test would thus be useful in assessing the clinical competence of students in nursing programs over a wide geographic area.

Four nurse-educators, three of them with expertise in maternity nursing and the fourth a nurse-researcher and expert in public health nursing and sociology, reviewed the film and validated the film content and nursing actions.

A tape recording of the film's sound track was transcribed into print. This written summary of the dialogue proved useful in the development of test questions and in recalling events depicted in the film without the need to see the film each time a question arose regarding content, sequence, or action. However, I did purchase the film in order to have it available for reference whenever necessary.

DEVELOPMENT OF THE TEST

The final multiple-choice paper-and-pencil test was developed in the following sequence. Spelling out in detail the steps taken in the development of this test serves a cautionary purpose. The process was lengthy and time-consuming, and one should not undertake such a venture without careful consideration of everything involved and, preferably, much experience in the area of test construction.

The first step was to generate the objectives of a typical unit on "care of the normal healthy woman during labor and delivery." An evaluation blueprint was then constructed, indicating those objectives that could be measured in a paper-and-pencil test and the taxonomic domain of each. The objectives that were psychomotor in nature later served as the basis for the development of the behaviors checklist discussed in Chapter 4. In some instances the objectives were classified as both cognitive and psychomotor since their attainment could probably be assessed in both ways.

The objectives could have been grouped into categories, that is, those dealing with assessment and those with observation. Instead they were designed to be sequential, in line with what a nurse would need to know or

---

*The 1976 edition of The American Journal of Nursing Co., 1976 Catalog of Audio Visuals listed five films on pediatric nursing and ten on obstetric nursing, exclusive of lectures on film.

do when a patient is admitted to the hospital in labor and to take care of the patient as she progresses through to delivery of her infant. The objectives generated for the unit under study and the taxonomic classification(s) of each of them are listed in Table 3-1.

Specifications for test content were defined in terms of gross content areas and levels of the cognitive domain exclusive of the lowest level, knowledge [4]. Items in the knowledge category tend to be easiest to write and are therefore likely to make up the bulk of most written tests. Since to test such items in a film does seem wasteful, an effort was made not to write any items for this level in this test. Bloom's *Taxonomy of Educational Objectives* [4] was used in developing one dimension of the blueprint, while the labor and delivery room component of the obstetric nursing course was used as the other. Although the blueprint was an essential step in the construction of the test, it was anticipated that it would probably need to be revised, depending upon the pool of test items that could be written. In allocating items in each of the content areas, major emphasis was given to those nursing needs of mothers and babies typically emphasized in nursing courses. For example, the woman in labor requires more nursing intervention over a longer period than does one in the recovery phase following delivery. And in this case, the major portion of the film was also devoted to the patient's labor; it was thus felt that more items could be written on the subject of labor.

One word about the synthesis and evaluation categories of the taxonomy: Reports by Bloom [4], Mandrillo [17], and Kropp and Stoker [14, p. 48] maintained that construction of multiple-choice items at these levels was fruitless. In spite of this, however, it was decided to include the two categories and attempt to construct some items at those levels.

Table 3-2 shows how many multiple-choice items were to be written for each level of the cognitive domain except knowledge in each of the content areas. A total of 60 items were decided on since that many questions of the multiple-choice type can be comfortably administered and answered in a one-hour period, assuming that approximately one minute is adequate for reading and responding to each. Although a time limit was imposed, the test was designed as a power test rather than a speed test, and, as such, every student had sufficient time to attempt to answer every question.

This kind of test blueprint differs from that commonly found in most textbooks on the subject. The taxonomy is usually omitted, listing objectives instead, but the subject matter dimension is generally included. If one were to analyze the objectives, however, they might very well fall into a hierarchy of the cognitive domain. The following example demonstrates that statement:

1. Applies principles of medical aseptic technique in the care of patients with communicable diseases
2. Understands facts and principles of medical aseptic technique in the care of patients with communicable diseases

Obviously objective 1 is higher in the taxonomy than objective 2.

Table 3-1. Evaluation Blueprint

Objectives for Unit on Care of the Normal Healthy Woman During Labor and Delivery	Domain Classification							
	Cognitive						Affective	Psychomotor
	Knowledge	Comprehension	Application	Analysis	Synthesis	Evaluation		
General								
Identifies the characteristics of a normal labor and delivery, relating each to the appropriate sciences		X						
Records and reports pertinent information, including maternal behavior, vital signs of the mother, fetal heart rate, character of contractions, signs and symptoms of labor, and so on								X
Gives anticipatory guidance to the laboring woman and her family							X	X
Establishes and maintains a constructive relationship with the patient and her family							X	
Indicates steps that can be taken to provide safe and effective nursing care to individual patients						X		
Collaborates with members of the health team in order to attain patient care goals								X
Supports the medical plan of care	X							X
Interprets medical explanations accurately to the patient and her family and in language appropriate for the individual								X
Identifies unsafe factors in the patient's environment and the measures appropriate for correcting them		X						X
Conforms to institutional and health department regulations for the protection of patients and personnel		X						X
Demonstrates effective organization of work habits with awareness of priorities					X			X
Adapts nursing procedures to meet the needs of individual patients, using general principles as well as those specific to the care of women in the intrapartal period		X						X
Describes the influence of culture on the individual during the birth process		X						
Describes physiological nutritional alterations associated with the intrapartal period	X or	X						
Adheres to policy regarding maintenance of hydration in women during the intrapartal period		X						X
Identifies physiological alterations of elimination in women during the intrapartal period		X						
Institutes measures to facilitate elimination in the patient during the intrapartal period		X						X

Table 3–1 (continued)

Objectives for Unit on Care of the Normal Healthy Woman During Labor and Delivery	Domain Classification — Cognitive						Affective	Psychomotor
	Knowledge	Comprehension	Application	Analysis	Synthesis	Evaluation	Affective	Psychomotor
Demonstrates manipulative skill and technical competence in caring for the patient during the intrapartal period								X
Early labor								
Differentiates true labor from false labor				X				
Describes the mental and physical changes that occur in primigravidas and multigravidas as labor approaches	X							
Describes presentations and positions of fetuses of differing sizes in relation to the maternal pelvis				X				
Labor								
Indicates measures likely to be used by the doctor for the laboring woman and their implications for nursing care			X					
Compares the effects of drugs commonly used with patients during labor and delivery, showing awareness of average doses and expected and untoward effects						X		
Assesses the progress and character of labor						X		
Describes the physiological and psychological symptoms characteristic of labor, including the average duration of each stage	X							
Identifies physical and emotional support measures that can be used by the nurse in each stage of labor to promote patient comfort					X			
Instructs the patient in appropriate breathing techniques during each stage of labor								X
Differentiates the course of labor for primigravidous women as compared with multigravidous women				X				
Describes the forces involved in labor	X							
Describes the mechanisms of labor	X							
Monitors vital signs of the mother and fetal heart rate using either conventional methods or electronic equipment								X
Assesses the emotional status of patients using both verbal and nonverbal cues						X		
Institutes measures to promote maximum relaxation during the intrapartal period								X
Encourages laboring women to use self-help techniques to promote relaxation, rest, and comfort								X

Table 3-1 (continued)

Objectives for Unit on Care of the Normal Healthy Woman During Labor and Delivery	Domain Classification							
	Cognitive							
	Knowledge	Comprehension	Application	Analysis	Synthesis	Evaluation	Affective	Psychomotor
Instructs husbands in measures to promote their wives' physical comfort and emotional security								X
Keeps the woman and her husband apprised of the progress of labor						X		X
Describes the characteristic emotional changes occurring in women during the intrapartal period	X							
Evaluates the reduction of tension in laboring women						X		
Predelivery								
Compares the effects of commonly used anesthetic agents and methods						X		
Describes the nursing implications in caring for laboring women receiving any of the commonly used anesthetics						X		
Birth								
Performs safely and effectively those procedures that must be done, according to hospital policy, for an infant before he is transferred from the delivery room to the nursery			X					X
Conducts an appraisal of the newborn infant using the Apgar scoring system								X
Interprets the significance of findings of Apgar score appraisal						X		X
Shows the infant to his mother in the delivery room prior to the infant's transfer to the nursery								X
Transfers the newborn infant from the delivery room to the nursery, following established institutional policies			X					X
Recovery phase								
Evaluates uterine tone and lochia in the first hour after delivery, intervening appropriately if indicated						X		X
Arranges for the new family to be together in the first hour after delivery, providing the hospital permits such an arrangement			X					X
Assists new parents in getting to know their infant								X
Assists the mother in helping her infant to nurse soon after delivery								X

Table 3–2. Original Blueprint of Specifications for Labor and Delivery Content and Cognitive Objectives[a]

	Content Based on Labor and Delivery Unit in Obstetric Nursing Course				
Cognitive Objective	Early Labor	Active Labor	Delivery	Recovery Phase	Initial Infant Care	Number of Items
Comprehension	2	2	1	1	1	7
Application	3	3	1	1	1	9
Analysis	5	5	1	1	1	13
Synthesis	5	5	2	2	1	15
Evaluation	5	5	2	2	2	16
Total	20	20	7	7	6	60

[a]Time: one hour; items: 60 four-option multiple-choice questions.

Thirty four-option multiple-choice questions based on the objectives covered in the film were written. A difficulty level of 50 percent was the aim for each question in order to "increase the variance of test scores and to increase the reliability of the test [24, p. 63]." Tinkelman [24, p. 63] and Lord and Novick [15] have stated that the difficulty of the individual item should be neither too hard nor too easy since questions of either type contribute little to test variance. For multiple-choice tests, Tinkelman [24, p. 64] says that the average uncorrected item difficulty should be a little easier than the 50 percent level with some dispersion of item difficulty. Thorndike and Hagen [23, p. 215] have stated that for four-option multiple-choice questions the average difficulty should be 74 percent, which would ". . . allow for the possibility of getting right answers by guessing." The difficulty level suggested also would ". . . yield a set of test scores that will be maximally useful to a teacher if he wants to discriminate levels of achievement among his students [23, pp. 49–50]." In the final selection of items, however, difficulty level is not the only criterion. Items must help the teacher to distinguish between the knowledgeable and unknowledgeable students. In addition, the content must represent adequate coverage of both subject matter and objectives [13; 23, pp. 49–50]. Since test questions with homogeneous options tend to be more difficult than those with heterogeneous ones, an attempt was made to keep the distracters homogeneous.

Validation of the questions was done by test constructors with expertise in maternity nursing. Other means of validation included obtaining support for the stem of the question when necessary, and ensuring the correct option and the negation of the distracters in current obstetrical textbooks and periodicals.

The next step after validation of the questions was deciding how to present them. Two methods were given serious consideration because of one advantage they shared—the ability to present questions related to the film content right after the event to be questioned, thus sooner than in the traditional paper-and-pencil test. The first method was to incorporate the questions into the film itself and stop the projector when they appeared. Although this technique posed some technical problems, most could have been solved by a competent film splicer. Also the projector would have to be left on to illuminate the questions while putting the room lights back on to enable students to mark their answer sheets. This stop-film technique, while not as impossible as it may sound, would probably work better with a shorter film and fewer questions. The other method considered was to use a slide projector for presentation of the questions, making administration slightly more complex. It was decided not to use either method since neither seemed to offer sufficient gain over the conventional written format. This decision would appear to be corroborated by the findings of Curtis and Kropp [10]; they state, in fact, that in some instances there is a loss of effectiveness. The final form of test presentation decided on is discussed below.

The first draft of 30 test questions was administered to two groups of students in one baccalaureate program. One group of students had had obstetric nursing while the other group had not. The grouping of the students in this way was an attempt to ascertain, if possible, whether the questions did in fact test obstetric nursing knowledge. (It is interesting to note that although the students who had not had obstetric nursing were the more interested of the two in seeing the film they were quite distressed when asked to answer the questions based on it, even though they had been told about the procedure beforehand.) On the basis of subsequent item analysis, revisions were made in those questions that were nondiscriminating, that is, those in which the correct answer to the question was selected more frequently by the lower-scoring students. Options were also modified when no one selected them.

The next draft of the test, containing an additional three questions, was administered to a group of six nurse-midwives and two obstetric nursing experts. A lengthy discussion of the items followed, and suggestions by the group for revision were later incorporated. Ideas were also presented that led to the development of an additional 18 questions. These questions were subsequently validated by the nurse-midwives and other consultants.

The third draft, now consisting of 51 items, was administered to 46 students in a baccalaureate program. The test was divided into two parts, a labor section and a delivery section. The students were shown the film twice, the first time straight through and the second in two parts. (The majority of students questioned after the administration of an early form of the test were overwhelmingly in favor of having the film immediately repeated.) Students took the first part of the test after seeing the first part of the film for the second time; the second part was taken after they saw that part of the film again. Administering parts of the test after the appropriate section of the film had been seen a second time was an attempt to minimize as much as possible the negative effects of memory and perception. By seeing the film once straight through, students would get the same input as if they were following a real patient in a clinical situation (considering, of course, the compression of events in a film in comparison to real time). Since some of the important events portrayed in the film are of such short duration, however, it was felt that a second exposure to the stimulus would increase retention.

A rather detailed set of instructions was developed in an attempt to standardize test administration as much as possible. The final form of the instructions is given on page 28. Following machine scoring of the IBM answer sheets, cards were keypunched for computer processing and item analysis data were obtained. Relatively minor revisions in the test questions were then made, primarily in those options not chosen by anyone.

DIRECTIONS FOR ADMINISTERING THE TEST
Preparing for Administration of the Test

1. As with other examinations during which no textbooks or aids are permitted in the testing room, students will be directed to deposit all such materials in an appropriate facility.
2. Scrap paper will be on each desk to permit note-taking.
3. The film will be ready for showing, with focus and sound adjusted.
4. Answer sheets, #2 pencils, and test booklets will be organized so that distribution at the appropriate time will be facilitated.

Administering the Test

The students will be read the following:

You are going to see a film called *Birth Day—Through the Eyes of the Mother,* which follows a pregnant woman from the time she is admitted to the hospital in labor through delivery of her baby. The film is thirty minutes long. In viewing the film, try to imagine yourself as an observer who is actually in the patient's room and charged with the responsibility of assessing the care the patient receives. You may take notes during the showing of the film, but do not let this activity interfere with your observation.

After you have seen the film through once, you will then immediately be shown the first part of the film again, that part dealing with the patient's admission and early labor. You will then answer some questions relating to the observations you have just made. After you have taken that short test, you will then be shown the next part of the film again, the portion dealing with the patient's active labor. You will then answer some questions which relate to that portion of the film. The last part of the film will then be shown, the part covering the delivery. Again, you will answer some questions, this time relating to the patient's delivery as well as some that pertain to the film as a whole.

The test booklets, answer sheets, and pencils will be distributed after you have seen the first part of the film for the second time, and more specific directions pertaining to the test will be given when the tests are distributed.

It is especially important that you not talk during the showings of the film nor, of course, when you take the test. Are there any questions?

WHEN TO STOP THE FILM

Stop the film for the first time when the doctor comes back into the patient's room and says: "What's happening here?"

Stop the film for the second time when the patient is being taken to the delivery room.

The fourth draft of 51 items was rearranged and now consisted of three parts: the first part concerned the patient's admission to the hospital and her early labor; the second concerned her active labor; and the third dealt with delivery of the infant and the film as a whole. This format was subsequently used for the final form of the test, although minor changes were made in the instructions to conform to the revisions in the test format.

The test was then administered to 17 baccalaureate students in another
school. As with the previous group, each part of the test was taken after
the respective part of the film had been seen for the second time.

Minor revisions were made in the test questions following study of the
new item analysis data. An additional nine items were also written in order
to provide a more representative sample of the subject matter. These new
items were also validated by the content experts and by means of current
literature, although they were not "tried out" prior to their inclusion in
the final form of the test.

The difficulty and discrimination indices of the items in the final form
of the test and the frequency distribution of these indices are given in
Table 3-3. The difficulty of an item is based on the proportion of examinees choosing the correct option. The ability of an item to discriminate
those students who scored high on the total test from those who got the
item wrong was computed for each item and is expressed as a biserial correlation. After all necessary data had been keypunched on cards, the
computer program computed the means, standard deviations, skewness,
kurtosis, part scores, subscores, and reliability coefficients for the test
parts and the total test. Students had been instructed to guess if they were
not sure of the correct answer, although cautioned against wild guessing;
the formula to correct for the effects of guessing had been utilized in all
phases of the development of the test. (This formula, for a test of four-
option questions, subtracts one-third of the wrong answers from those
scored correctly [23, p. 250] .) When examining the data, consideration
should be given to the sample size—267 students—since small n's tend to

Table 3-3. Difficulty and Discrimination Indices and Frequency Distributions of Items in Final Form of the Test

Difficulty		Discrimination	
p	No. of Items	Biserial[a]	No. of Items
		Below .00	2
		.00–.04	2
		.05–.09	4
.10–.19	3	.10–.14	3
.20–.29	9	.15–.19	6
.30–.39	6	.20–.24	8
.40–.49	4	.25–.29	12
.50–.59	9	.30–.34	9
.60–.69	10	.35–.39	7
.70–.79	10	.40–.44	1
.80–.89	7	.45–.49	3
.90–.99	2	.50–.54	3
Total	60	Total	60

p = Proportion of examinees who chose the correct answer.
[a]Discriminating ability of the correct option.

distort item statistics. Another probable factor was the relative emphasis placed on the content of the question by the instructor.

The next step in the development of the test was to have the subject matter experts code the items into two areas: those items for which the stimulus of the film was necessary and those that could probably be answered without seeing the film. The 28 questions in the former category were designated Subscore A,* while the remaining 32 questions became Subscore B.* It would have been ideal to have all of the items depend upon the stimulus of the film, but since that was not possible, the Subscore B items were included to extend the sample of content.

The items were then coded according to the cognitive levels listed in the test specifications (see Table 3-4), a task that proved surprisingly complex. What may be application for one student, for example, may simply be recall for another, depending upon his or her experience, mode of learning, and recency of experience. A great deal depends on the wording of the question; for example, a student who has seen a doctor's order for reverse isolation technique for a patient with leukemia or who has cared for such a patient may merely be recalling information about such an order, while another student knows only that patients with leukemia are extremely susceptible to infection and deduces that protection from pathogenic organisms is necessary.

Because of the difficulty encountered in coding the items, three experienced test constructors were asked to assist. Examples of behaviorial terms and objectives devised by Gronlund [11] were distributed to each of the coders who then worked independently. Unanimous agreement was reached for only 33 percent, or 20, of the items. For another 33 percent there was agreement among two of the coders and myself. Since consensus by at least three coders was not attained for the remaining 20 items, I took responsibility for the final decision, based chiefly on three qualifications: (1) prior experience with undergraduate nursing students and their curriculum, (2) familiarity with film content, and (3) the knowledge that students had probably not been taught the specific content contained in the item; this last qualification was especially significant at the application level. Since the filmed clinical simulation of a previously studied situation was new to all students, items relating to content in the film, in general, had to test for the *application* of knowledge rather than the lower levels of the cognitive domain, thus requiring students to make judgments from the cues provided.

Two factors probably related to the difficulty or ease of coding items were how long ago and how many times the film was seen. Two coders saw the film once, and one saw it twice, and I saw it approximately 20 times. As a result, occasional clarification of events in the film were needed by the three assisting coders.

*Subscore A items: 1, 2, 3, 7, 11, 15, 18, 19, 26, 28, 29, 31, 33, 34, 36–38, 41–45, 51, 53, 56–59; Subscore B items: 4–6, 8–10, 12–14, 16, 17, 20–25, 27, 30, 32, 35, 39, 40, 46–50, 52, 54, 55, 60.

This difficulty in coding was not unexpected since others had reported similar problems [7; 14, p. 21] . In view of what, for example, Bormuth [5, p. 77] says—that ". . . correct responses to test items are inherently ambiguous, for it can never be shown conclusively that the student has indeed learned the capability the item is designed to test"—it can be inferred that coding ultimately rests with the test developer [5, p. 11] . It is probably more difficult for someone to code items in a standardized test than it is for a teacher to code his or her own test; however, an instructor can analyze previously developed tests by using an already existing coding system, adapting one to his or her own needs, or creating one to meet a particular need. The difficulty is particularly acute in the case of items based on a simulation, since the factors of memory and visual perception are also operative.

The coding of items into the content categories posed relatively little difficulty, perhaps because most of the content was quite clear-cut. On occasion items could be equally applicable to another content area, for example, early labor or active labor. Other items were so general in nursing content that another area—miscellaneous—had to be added to the blueprint for items falling into that category.

Since the number of items at each cognitive level and in each content area differed from the blueprint previously prepared, it was necessary to alter the test specifications to conform to what the test now contained. The original time limit had been set at one hour, but since the film is thirty minutes long and is shown twice, the overall time period was changed to two hours to include viewing time.

As has been mentioned previously, because of the difficulty in writing multiple-choice items at the higher cognitive levels, there were no items assessing attainment of objectives at the synthesis level. There were nine items at the evaluation process level and 21 at the analysis level, a full 50 percent of the total test. Certain portions of the film—mainly the recovery phase after delivery and initial infant care—were so deficient in testable content due to the brevity of presentation that very few test items could be written. The revised test blueprint is shown on Table 3–4.

Because the film on which the test is based was readily available, it was necessary to establish that the students had not seen it in conjunction with their obstetric nursing course. If students had seen the film and if their instructors had discussed its numerous deficiencies and merits with them, it would have influenced and invalidated the test results. (Such a situation is unlikely to occur, however, when a film is developed for the specific purpose of providing the stimulus for a test, in which case the film content can be kept secure.)

In order to standardize the conditions of administration to the maximum degree, I personally administered the test at all four of the participating schools (as well as at the preliminary tryouts).

In final form, the test consisted of 60 four-option multiple-choice questions divided into three parts and was prepared by photo-offset process.

Table 3–4. Revised and Final Blueprint of Specifications for Labor and Delivery Content and Cognitive Objectives[a]

Cognitive Objective	Content Based on Labor and Delivery Unit in Obstetric Nursing Course						Number of Items
	Early Labor[b]	Active Labor[b]	Delivery	Recovery Phase	Initial Infant Care	Miscellaneous[c]	
Knowledge	5	1	1	1	2	3	13
Comprehension	0	3	0	1	1	3	8
Application	4	2	2	0	0	1	9
Analysis	6	6	3	1	0	5	21
Synthesis	0	0	0	0	0	0	0
Evaluation	1	4	0	0	1	3	9
Total	16	16	6	3	4	15	60

[a]Time: two hours (includes one hour for viewing the film); items: 60 four-option multiple choice questions.
[b]Occasional items pertaining to both early and active labor could be categorized in either area.
[c]Includes items pertaining to obstetric nursing but that are general in nature.

Each part was sealed off from the next, and the students were instructed not to go on to the next part of the test until told to do so. All instructions were printed on the first page of the test booklet. The final form of the test is reproduced at the end of this chapter (see page 46).

TEST CHARACTERISTICS

A potential test user must be given information about numerous test characteristics in order for him or her to assess its usefulness for a given purpose. Among the characteristics described below are item and test difficulty, the difficulty level of the various test parts, and discrimination indices. Also to be discussed, separately, are the two criteria by which the quality of any test can be judged: reliability and validity. Evidence of several kinds of validity will be presented.

Item Difficulty

The proportion of examinees who chose the correct answer reflects the difficulty of an item and is shown for the final form of the test in Tables 3-3 and 3-5. While there are several easy and several difficult items, almost one-half are between 50 and 79 percent. Item difficulty is unrelated to the cognitive process level, a not unexpected finding. For example, item 7, an analysis item, had a difficulty level of 64.8 percent while lower level item 2, a comprehension item, had a difficulty level of 42.3 percent.

Mean difficulty and discrimination indices were computed for the 30 items at the lower cognitive levels—knowledge, comprehension, and application—and for the 30 items at the higher cognitive levels—analysis and evaluation. There was very little difference between the two categories, as is shown in these results; if anything, the items at the higher cognitive levels were easier.

	Mean Difficulty Index	Mean Discrimination Index
Lower cognitive levels	.541	.263
Higher cognitive levels	.559	.261

Difficulty of the Test and Its Parts

Table 3-6 reveals that the difficulty of each of the five individual scores obtained (51.8 percent to 59.8 percent) differs little from the difficulty of the test as a whole, 55.0 percent. Part 3 was the easiest one of the three, with a difficulty of 59.8 percent. At 56.8 percent, the easier of the two subscore parts was Subscore A, the items that required seeing the film.

Discrimination Indices

Biserial correlations were computed for each item and indicate the relationship between the item and the test part or between the item and the total score, specifically the discriminating ability of the correct answer. Table 3-3 shows the frequency distributions of the discrimination indices and that 29 items had biserial correlations ranging from .20 to .34; 14 items had biserial coefficients ranging from .35 to .54. Of the remaining

Table 3-5. Item Analysis and Code for Final Form of Test

Item No.	Correct Option	Sub-score[a]	Difficulty Index	Discrimination Index— Biserial	Cognitive Level	Subject Matter Area
1	3	A	.809	.324	Analysis	Early labor
2	4	A	.423	.532	Comprehension	Miscellaneous
3	1	A	.322	.264	Application	Early labor
4	4	B	.472	.164	Evaluation	Early labor
5	4	B	.221	.274	Analysis	Early labor
6	3	B	.876	.049	Application	Early labor
7	2	A	.648	.294	Analysis	Delivery
8	2	B	.371	.376	Knowledge	Miscellaneous
9	3	B	.270	.121	Knowledge	Early labor
10	1	B	.734	.213	Knowledge	Early labor
11	4	A	.288	.352	Application	Early labor
12	3	B	.524	.210	Analysis	Early labor
13	2	B	.116	.261	Knowledge	Early labor
14	4	B	.727	.357	Analysis	Early labor
15	4	A	.659	.213	Analysis	Early labor
16	2	B	.509	.263	Knowledge	Early labor
17	4	B	.655	.085	Knowledge	Early labor
18	3	A	.921	.341	Analysis	Early labor
19	4	A	.288	.340	Application	Early labor
20	1	B	.206	.318	Analysis	Active labor
21	1	B	.348	.277	Analysis	Active labor
22	1	B	.307	.534	Comprehension	Active labor
23	3	B	.727	.243	Comprehension	Active labor
24	1	B	.903	.335	Comprehension	Miscellaneous

25	B	.805	.360	Application	Active labor
26	A	.303	.486	Evaluation	Active labor
27	B	.562	.281	Comprehension	Active labor
28	A	.367	.169	Evaluation	Active labor
29	A	.663	.185	Analysis	Active labor
30	B	.434	.243	Comprehension	Miscellaneous
31	A	.715	.240	Analysis	Active labor
32	B	.176	.182	Application	Active labor
33	A	.730	.303	Evaluation	Miscellaneous
34	A	.596	.362	Analysis	Active labor
35	B	.266	.353	Knowledge	Active labor
36	A	.745	-.008	Evaluation	Active labor
37	A	.547	.328	Evaluation	Active labor
38	A	.206	-.048	Analysis	Active labor
39	B	.670	.466	Application	Delivery
40	B	.213	.268	Knowledge	Delivery
41	A	.607	.318	Analysis	Delivery
42	A	.678	.249	Analysis	Delivery
43	A	.768	.154	Knowledge	Infant care
44	A	.524	.402	Comprehension	Infant care
45	A	.738	.133	Evaluation	Infant care
46	B	.813	.059	Comprehension	Recovery
47	B	.869	.080	Knowledge	Infant care
48	B	.124	.460	Analysis	Recovery
49	B	.876	.299	Knowledge	Recovery
50	B	.577	.261	Knowledge	Miscellaneous
51	A	.603	.352	Analysis	Miscellaneous
52	B	.689	.287	Analysis	Miscellaneous
53	A	.251	.526	Analysis	Miscellaneous
54	B	.577	.147	Analysis	Miscellaneous

Table 3-5 (continued)

Item No.	Correct Option	Sub-score[a]	Difficulty Index	Discrimination Index— Biserial	Cognitive Level	Subject Matter Area
55	3	B	.749	.088	Knowledge	Miscellaneous
56	4	A	.652	.239	Analysis	Miscellaneous
57	2	A	.899	.326	Evaluation	Miscellaneous
58	3	A	.416	.167	Application	Delivery
59	2	A	.532	.005	Evaluation	Miscellaneous
60	3	B	.723	.288	Application	Miscellaneous

[a]Subscore A = items that cannot be answered without seeing the film; subscore B = items that can probably be answered without seeing the film.

Table 3-6. Mean Difficulty and Discrimination Indices of Final Form of Test and Its Parts

Test Part	No. of Items	Mean Difficulty Index	Mean Discrimination Index—r_{bis}
Part 1	19	.518	.265
Part 2	18	.522	.288
Part 3	23	.598	.240
Subscore A[a]	28	.568	.270
Subscore B[b]	32	.534	.256
Total	60	.550	.264

[a]Those items that cannot be answered without seeing the film.
[b]Those items that can probably be answered without seeing the film.

17 items, two had negative biserial coefficients, and 15 had a low discriminating power, if one considers a biserial correlation of below .20 as low. In spite of the low correlations, however, the mean discrimination index of the total test was .264 (see Table 3-6). Table 3-5 gives the biserial correlation for each item.

Correlation Between Test Parts

Each one of the five test parts was correlated with each of the four others as well as with the total test (Table 3-7). Of the three parts, Part 3 correlated to the greatest degree with Part 1 (.356), with Subscore B (.621), and also with the total test (.756). The correlation of Subscore A with the total test was similar to that between Subscore B and the total test. It should be noted that Part 3 contained more items than Parts 1 and 2, and Subscore B contained more items than did Subscore A. These correlations between scores on parts of the test and the total test are inflated because the items used for the total test scores include the items used for scores on the separate parts of the test. Attention also needs to be drawn to the fact that subscore items are interspersed throughout the three test parts, as can be seen in Table 3-10, so that subscore-part correlations are also spuriously inflated (see footnote in Table 3-7).

Reliability

An instrument's consistency of measurement can be estimated in a number of ways. The method used for this test, one of internal consistency, employed the Kuder-Richardson Formula 20 (KR20). Guilford and Fruchter [12, p. 416, 419] state that KR20 is the most appropriate estimate of internal consistency for power tests. Another reason for my use of KR20 was Magnusson's [16] point that ". . . KR20 gives the mean of the distribution of coefficients we should obtain if we were to compute every possible split-half coefficient for the test."

The reliability coefficients, shown in Table 3-8, obtained for the five test parts ranged from .621 for Part 2 to .697 for Subscore A (the items that required viewing the film). All of the part scores and both subscores were

Table 3-7. Correlation Coefficients Between Test Parts and the Total Test[a]
(N = 267)

Test Part	Part 1	Part 2	Part 3	Subscore A	Subscore B	Total Test
Part 1	—	.195	.356	.545	.603	.703
Part 2	.195	—	.327	.599	.580	.716
Part 3	.356	.327	—	.595	.621	.756
Subscore A	.545	.599	.595	—	.337	.811
Subscore B	.603	.580	.621	.337	—	.820
Total test	.703	.716	.756	.811	.820	—

[a]Correlations are spuriously high between test parts and the total because the parts are included in the total. Also, subscore items are intermixed in all parts.

Table 3-8. Reliability Coefficients and Standard Errors of Measurement for Final Form of Test and Its Parts

Test Part	No. of Items	KR20	S.E.$_m$
Part 1	19	.644	1.84
Part 2	18	.621	1.82
Part 3	23	.622	2.03
Subscore A[a]	28	.697	2.31
Subscore B[b]	32	.684	2.38
Total	60	.764	3.35

[a]Those items that cannot be answered without seeing the film.
[b]Those items that can probably be answered without seeing the film.
KR20 = Kuder-Richardson Formula 20; S.E.$_m$ = standard error of measurement.

lower than the total test score, which was .764. Magnusson [16] states that "The more homogeneous the items are, the greater the numerical value of KR20 will be for a given number of items in the test." Guilford and Fruchter [12, p. 418] say that all of the formulas for estimating internal consistency, exclusive of test-retest administrations, probably underestimate the reliability of a test and that, in particular, the KR20 "gives an underestimate when there is wide dispersion of item difficulties."

In partial explanation of the low reliability coefficients, one should consider how heterogeneous the test is. Items deal with psychological aspects, pharmacological content, pathological facts, nutritional aspects, and other material dealing with obstetric nursing, and, as such, one would expect that the reliability coefficients would be lower than for a test exclusively on, for example, the pharmacological aspects of patient care. Because of this heterogeneity, the use of the odd-even method for calculating reliability would probably have yielded lower reliability coefficients.

Since no test is a perfect measuring instrument, the standard error of measurement was computed for each test part and for the total test (Table 3–8). They ranged from 1.82 for Part 2 to 2.38 for Subscore B. For the total test, the standard error of measurement was 3.35.

Validity

Three kinds of validity will be discussed: content, construct, and concurrent validity. No attempt was made to gather evidence related to predictive validity. It should be noted that some authorities [8, 21] consider criterion-related validity as one of the three major types of validity (the other two being content and construct validity) with predictive and concurrent validity subsumed. The ability to predict a student's clinical performance from the test score would be a type of criterion-related validity.

CONTENT VALIDITY

According to *Standards for Educational and Psychological Tests and Manuals* [1], content validation is usually of primary importance for an achievement test. Content validity was obtained for this test by subject-matter experts, in particular nurse-midwives, nurses knowledgeable in maternity nursing care and in test construction, and through the use of current obstetric textbooks and periodicals. The last-named was used to (1) support the information presented in the stem of the question when necessary, (2) support the correct answer, and (3) negate the distracters.

All the experts agreed that the test content reflected information presented in the film and that it was representative of the universe of content in a unit on the care of normal healthy women during labor and delivery. A teacher-made test blueprint for the same unit might have included more, but this particular test was limited because of what was already in the film. Because of the limited number of items based on film content that could be developed, the sample of test questions from the universe of content was deliberately extended, chiefly to be more representative of the unit.

CONSTRUCT AND CONCURRENT VALIDITY

Construct and concurrent validity will be discussed together since there is an area of overlap. It was hypothesized that students scoring high on the criterion behaviors checklist (the performance tool discussed in Chap. 4, p. 64) would also score high on this test. The same kind of relationship was hypothesized to exist between the National League for Nursing achievement test. Content validity was obtained for this test by subject-esis could not be tested at this time since none of the schools in the sample used any of the League achievement tests.

Anastasi [2] states that to some degree the internal consistency of a subtest contributes to the establishment of a test's construct validity. In the instance of Subscore A, the items requiring the viewing of the film, scores correlated higher with the performance scores obtained on the behaviors checklist than did those from Subscore B. It had been theorized that the students who obtained the high scores on the test were identifying the components of poor or inadequate nursing practice that were depicted in the film and tested in Subscore A questions and would therefore be unlikely to commit the same kinds of errors in their own practice. The correlations were so low, however, that this theory was not tenable from a statistical frame of reference.

Another approach for testing the relationship between test scores and performance scores (as determined by the behaviors checklist) was to correlate the top 25 percent checklist scores with the top 25 percent test scores and the bottom 25 percent checklist scores with the same bottom percent test scores. This method yielded correlations not unlike those obtained using the total.

The 30 items in the test at the highest levels of cognition—the analysis and evaluation levels—were examined in terms of mean difficulty and discrimination indices. It had been anticipated that the difficulty level of items would be unrelated to their cognitive level but that the mean discrimination index of the higher cognitive level questions would better distinguish knowledgeable students from those less knowledgeable. The former expectation held up, but the latter one did not, since the indices differed only slightly (higher in both instances) from those computed for the total test.

TEST SCORES
Test items were scored dichotomously, that is, the student either got the answer right or wrong. No credit was given for distracters, although some tests have been designed to weight options in order of correctness. The formula to correct for guessing—substracting one-third of the wrong answers from the number of right ones—was employed, since the test was composed of four-option multiple-choice questions.

Part Scores
The first 19 items in the test (Part 1) were answered after the students had seen the first part of the film, dealing with the patient's admission to the hospital and her early labor, for the second time. The mean corrected score for all students was 6.81, or approximately 36 percent, with a standard deviation of 3.09 (Table 3-9).

The next 18 items compose Part 2 of the test and were answered by the students after they had seen the middle part of the film, relating to the patient's active labor, for the second time. In this part students also answered approximately 36 percent of the items correctly. Table 3-9 shows that the mean corrected score was 6.56, with a standard deviation of 2.96.

The remainder of the test, the last 23 items, was taken after students had seen the end of the film for the second time. Items in this part, Part 3, dealt with the delivery of the baby as well as the film as a whole. The mean corrected score was 10.65, with a standard deviation of 3.31. Students answered approximately 46 percent of these items correctly, indicating that Part 3 was the easiest part of the test.

Table 3-9. Means, Standard Deviations, Skewness, and Kurtosis for Test and Its Parts

Test Part	No. of Items	Mean	S.D.	Skewness	Kurtosis
Part 1	19	6.81	3.09	.34	2.54
Part 2	18	6.56	2.96	.11	2.82
Part 3	23	10.65	3.31	−.02	2.50
Subscore A[a]	28	11.90	4.20	−.10	2.94
Subscore B[b]	32	12.14	4.23	.40	3.09
Total	60	24.01	6.89	.25	2.89

[a]Those items that cannot be answered without seeing the film.
[b]Those items that can probably be answered without seeing the film.
S.D. = standard deviation.

Of the three test parts, the one with the greatest degree of skewness was Part 1 at .34, a moderate degree of positive skewing. Skewness, a measure that indicates the symmetry of a distribution, normally "varies within the limits of ±3 [9]."

Another indication of the distribution of a sample is kurtosis, which is the "degree of steepness of the middle part of the distribution [12, pp. 158-159]"; a normal curve has a kurtosis of 3.0. Part 2 was most meso-kurtic at 2.82. Table 3-9 shows the degrees of skewness and kurtosis for the five test parts.

Subscores

The items in the test were coded into two areas: Subscore A (28 items), those that cannot be answered without seeing the film; and Subscore B (32 items), those that can probably be answered without the stimulus of the film. Corrected for guessing, the mean number of items answered correctly for Subscore A was 11.90, approximately 43 percent of the items, and the standard deviation was 4.20; the mean for Subscore B was 12.14, approximately 38 percent of the items, and the standard deviation was 4.23 (Table 3-9). Also included in Table 3-9 are the measures of skewness and kurtosis. The greatest deviation from normal is that for Subscore B, for which the skewness was .40, which is a moderate degree of skewing to the right. The kurtosis is 3.09, which indicates the relative normalcy of the curve since a mesokurtic distribution is 3.0.

Subscore questions are distributed throughout all three parts of the test: Part 1, 8 items from Subscore A and 11 items from Subscore B; in Part 2, 8 items from Subscore A and 10 from Subscore B; Part 3, 12 items from Subscore A and 11 from Subscore B. Subscore A items constitute 28.6 percent of the items in Parts 1 and 2 and 42.8 percent of those in Part 3. Subscore B items are more evenly dispersed throughout the test, making up 34.4 percent of the items in Parts 1 and 3 and 31.2 percent of those in Part 2. Table 3-10 shows the numbers and percentages of item distribution.

Table 3-10. Number and Percentage of Items from Each Subscore in Each Test Part

	Subscore A		Subscore B	
Test Part	No. of Items	%	No. of Items	%
Part 1	8	28.6	11	34.4
Part 2	8	28.6	10	31.2
Part 3	12	42.8	11	34.4
Total	28	100.0	32	100.0

Total Test Scores

The total test score was based on the 60 test items, corrected for guessing or chance success. The total sample showed a range of 37 points, from the lowest score of 7 to the highest one of 44. The mean of the total group was 24.01, or approximately 40 percent of the items, with a standard deviation of 6.89. School means ranged from 21.20 to 30.38 and the standard deviations from 5.82 to 7.29. Table 3–11 shows the sample size in each school and gives the means, ranges of scores, and standard deviations for each as well as for the total group.

The degree of skewness in the distribution of scores for the total test was .25, a slight piling up of the scores to the left, indicating that a rather high number of the items were relatively difficult for the examinees. At 2.89, the sampling distribution of the total scores was quite mesokurtic. This finding is further substantiated by the size of the standard deviation for the total group. Table 3–9 shows the degrees of skewness and kurtosis for the total test as well as for its parts.

Item Omission Rate

The mean number of items not answered per examinee ranged from .03 for Parts 1 and 2 to .10 for the total test. This finding indicates that students followed the directions, in which they were told to attempt to answer all questions and to guess if they had any idea as to the correct answer but to avoid wild guessing. It also supports the allocation of time for test-taking and the contention that the test was indeed a power test rather than a speed one.

DISCUSSION OF THE TEST RESULTS AND SOME RECOMMENDATIONS

Many points about the findings have already been discussed, but further elaboration and discussion seem indicated. The reliability coefficient obtained for Subscore A, those items for which seeing the film is necessary, is higher (.697) than that for Subscore B. This may be due to the fact that those items are more homogeneous than those in Subscore B. It should also be noted that there are fewer items in Subscore A, and if the number

Table 3-11. Range of Scores, Mean Scores, and Standard Deviations for Four Sample Schools on Final Form of Test

Variable	School				Total Sample
	1	2	3	4	
Range of scores	11–40	7–37	7–39	21–44	7–44
Mean score	24.68	21.20	26.40	30.38	24.01
Standard deviation	5.82	5.89	7.29	6.12	6.89
Sample size	66	127	40	34	267

of items in that category had been increased, it would probably have yielded an even higher reliability coefficient. Therefore if this method were to be replicated in the future, it would be advisable to have more items that are directly dependent upon the stimulus of the film.

The KR20 reliability coefficient for Part 2 was lower than that for any of the three subtests and two subscores. One reason was undoubtedly the number of items, only 18. Conversely, the reliability coefficient for the total test was higher (.764) than for any of its components, again due in part to the number of items, in this case 60.

In attempting to establish the relative strength of the reliability coefficient obtained for the total test, the KR20 reliability coefficient for an obstetric nursing test of the State Board Test Pool Examination was used. It was .71. Although given in a 1971 article [18], the coefficient offered may have been several years old, and that fact should be borne in mind in any comparison. In the several years prior to 1971, there was a change in the number of items included in the obstetric nursing test from approximately 120 to approximately 90, which is the current practice. (The number of items included each year differs slightly.) A difference of 30 items, as is well known, can substantially influence the magnitude of the reliability coefficient obtained. What was reported may have been for a test of about 120 items, so that it is reasonable to assume that the reliability coefficient for a 90-item test would have been lower. If, however, one assumes that the reliability coefficient of .71 is for a 90-item test, then the higher (though not tremendous) reliability coefficient of .76 for the 60-item test under discussion deserves further consideration. Bearing in mind the large number of candidate scores used in computing the KR20 for the State Board Test Pool Examination and the small number of students used for the movie test, it is necessary to consider the possibility that other factors may also be influencing the internal consistency determination of this test. Perhaps one consideration should be the method of presenting the patient situation—the film—as compared with the verbal and therefore static descriptions used in the State Board Test Pool Examination. It is conceivable that examinees who have difficulty in interpreting the written word may have less trouble with visual or aural presentations, or both. Perhaps there is less ambiguity with the motion picture presentation.

A factor that certainly could have affected the level of difficulty of the test is the lack of sufficient clinical experience in a labor and delivery situation. The students who took this test had an absolute minimum of experience with women in labor, and unfortunately that situation seems to be universal. Only by being able to observe and care for women in labor can the student apply what she has learned in class and from her readings. For many students the first experience of a labor and delivery is so emotionally charged that little or no learning takes place. It would seem that more experience in that situation is essential but how to accomplish that aim is beyond the scope of this book. The film used in this study, however, which shows a real patient's labor and delivery, can complement actual clinical experience.

The test could be used with undergraduate nursing students, graduate students in obstetric nursing, or with nurse-midwifery students as a teaching tool rather than as an evaluation tool, with appropriate follow-up discussions by a qualified obstetric instructor. Its use in such a way would serve to supplement clinical experience; its use as both a pre- and posttest would be one means of evaluating gains students have made after their obstetric nursing experience. With minor modifications, the test might also prove useful as a self-study or self-assessment tool for all levels of nurses, undergraduates as well as graduates, its use with the latter being perhaps in conjunction with in-service education programs.

If one wants to use the test as presented, a word or two of caution is offered. To begin with, faculty should review each question in terms of both the correct answer and the distracters. If they do not agree with the correct answer given or feel that one or more of the distracters is too close to being correct, revisions should be made before the test is given. In addition, several of the items had negative biserial correlations and some others had low ones. These items should definitely be revised before use.

Any additional items based on film content that can be written should be included. It would be an inefficient use of time, however, to write additional items that do not require the film in order to answer them. (I certainly do not think that I exhausted the possibilities for questions!)

Prior to being used for purposes of assessing a student's knowledge and perhaps assigning a grade based on the student's performance, the revised test should be administered to a group of students comparable to those who will ultimately take it. In this instance, no grade should be assigned, and the students should be apprised of the purpose behind their taking the test.

A major problem encountered in construction of the test described in this chapter was that it was extremely time-consuming, more so than the usual paper-and-pencil test, and frequent viewings of the film in early stages were required to master the content. Even content validation by subject-matter experts required more time since they had to see the film more than one time in order to state with any degree of assurance what was or was not presented and the inferences that could be drawn from the cues presented. If, however, one were to construct a test based on a film that had been made to a predetermined plan, the test construction phase might be slightly less expensive in terms of time, although there would still be a lot of time involved in designing and making the film. One reason for the decrease in test construction time is that the content would already have been decided on and built into the film.

A Nursing Test Based on a Filmed Clinical Situation in Labor and Delivery

Instructions: The questions in this test are based on the content of the film you have just seen—"Birth Day—Through the Eyes of the Mother." The questions are to be answered on the basis of what you remember having seen and heard in the film.

There is only one type of question in this test, multiple choice with four possible answers. Select the *ONE* best answer for each question *and* ALL of the four choices offered. If you are not sure of the answer, a guess may aid you, since your score will be the number of right answers.

Use a No. 2 pencil for marking your answer sheet. Blacken the space for the answer you have selected. For example, if you select option number 4 for question 1, your answer sheet will look like this:

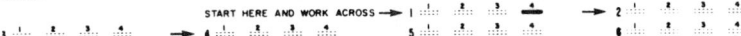

It is important that only *one* space be blackened for each question. Erase any stray marks you may make on the answer sheet.

The test will be administered in 3 parts. Each part will be taken after you have seen the section of the film that deals with the content of the questions which follow. You will have approximately 1 minute for each question. The last few questions in the test are general in nature, pertaining to the film as a whole.

If you finish before time is called, please remain quietly in your seat. Do *NOT* break the seal of the next section until told to do so.

In the boxed-in area of your answer sheet, please enter your name and school. This information is essential in order to compute the necessary statistical tests, although individuals and schools will remain anonymous in the final report.

Part 1
You will have 20 minutes to take this part of the test.

1. The nurse asked Maureen a question that was based on the assumption that Maureen
   1. had attended an antepartal clinic.
   2. was anxious about the outcome of the pregnancy.
   3. had been timing her contractions.
   4. was knowledgeable about what to expect in subsequent stages of labor.

2. During Maureen's admission, she talked about her reactions to Jean, the nurse who admitted her. Although Maureen didn't do so, she could justifiably have said,
   1. "It was nice to know that I wouldn't be alone during labor."
   2. "She was so petite, I thought I'd break her arm if I grabbed it."
   3. "Her explanation of everything to me was really great."
   4. "I didn't hear all that she said because her voice was so low pitched."

3. In relation to her own apparel, the admitting nurse should most certainly have
   1. removed her rings.
   2. worn her nurse's cap.
   3. been wearing her name pin.
   4. covered her scrub dress with a doctor's gown.

46

4. The nurse asked Maureen all of the following questions shortly after her admission. While all of the questions would be useful in establishing a nursing care plan, which one could justifiably have been postponed?
   1. "Have you been exposed recently to a communicable disease?"
   2. "Are you leaking any fluid?"
   3. "How much weight did you gain during your pregnancy?"
   4. "Do you expect to breast- or bottle-feed your baby?"

5. Which of these occurrences soon after Maureen was admitted would probably have *DIMINISHED* her confidence in the personnel?
   1. The nurse did not immediately notify the doctor of Maureen's arrival on the unit.
   2. Neither a doctor nor a nurse stayed with Maureen continuously.
   3. No one provided Maureen with information about the infant's condition.
   4. Maureen was asked the same questions by both the nurse and the doctor.

6. Maureen joked about the fact that she had been told what to expect in the hospital. What was probably the purpose of that behavior?
   1. To convey to personnel that she would cooperate with them.
   2. To get hospital staff to like her.
   3. To relieve her own anxiety.
   4. To demonstrate to pregnant women who would see the film that hospitalization was not a traumatic experience.

7. The doctor seemed to make several assumptions in relation to Maureen's labor and delivery. Which of them was most apparent?
   1. That Maureen was going to have a larger-than-average baby.
   2. That Maureen was going to have anesthesia.
   3. That Maureen's intrapartum course was going to be prolonged.
   4. That Maureen was going to require medication only at the end of the first stage of labor.

8. Maureen told the doctor that she hadn't gained any more weight since she started taking a diuretic and restricting the use of salt in her diet as prescribed. Which of these understandings, if any, about the use of the two measures to control weight gain during a normal pregnancy is accurate?
   1. They are commonly recommended because side effects rarely occur.
   2. They are medically controversial.
   3. The use of diuretics is considered to be safe and effective, but salt restriction is generally contraindicated.
   4. None of the above.

9. Maureen, referring to her cervical dilatation, asked the doctor how she was progressing. He replied, "Two centimeters." Which of these understandings about complete cervical dilatation in normal primigravidas is accurate?
   1. Effacement occurs before the onset of true labor, while cervical dilatation is dependent upon true labor contractions.
   2. Effacement precedes cervical dilatation, and the total process takes about 6 to 10 hours.
   3. Cervical dilatation occurs simultaneously with effacement and takes about 12 to 16 hours.
   4. Cervical dilatation precedes effacement, with the total process taking about 8 to 12 hours.

10. Prior to the perineal shave, in which position was Maureen placed?
    1. Lithotomy.
    2. Knee-chest.
    3. Trendelenburg's.
    4. Sims'.

11. The nurse explained several purposes of the perineal shave to Maureen. Which of these purposes should the nurse have added?
    1. To better visualize the area.
    2. To prevent hair from getting into the stitches.
    3. To provide a surgically clean field.
    4. To facilitate care of the area.

12. While Maureen was being shaved it would have been desirable for the nurse to say,
    1. "Although you will experience some discomfort when the hair grows back, shaving is a necessary procedure."
    2. "Women usually complain of a tickling sensation as the hair regrows, but it shouldn't pose any great problems for you."
    3. "It's common to be embarrassed because the shaving involves a private area, but it will help to promote the safety of the birth process."
    4. "We're pretty lucky not having to shave every day, aren't we?"

13. The nurse wore gloves when shaving Maureen. Which of these understandings is accurate about the practice of wearing gloves when shaving the perineum of a patient such as Maureen?
    1. They should be worn.
    2. They are unnecessary.
    3. They are worn when there is a leakage of amniotic fluid.
    4. They should certainly be worn if the patient's personal hygiene is poor.

14. Maureen made several comments in relation to the enema she was about to have. Which comment, if Maureen had made it, would indicate that the nurse did *NOT* prepare her adequately for the enema?
    1. "I thought I was going to drop the baby."
    2. "I had an enema as a child, but I've had none since then."
    3. "I won't be able to hold the fluid if I have a contraction."
    4. "I don't understand why an enema is so important."

15. The nurse's approach to Maureen while she was in labor appeared to be based on Maureen's
    1. socioeconomic status.
    2. prior experience with nurses and doctors.
    3. acceptance of the nurse as a helping person.
    4. preparation for childbirth.

16. When timing Maureen's contractions, the nurse's hand should have been
    1. cupped with the fingers extended.
    2. over the uterine fundus.
    3. moved from side to side across the lower abdomen.
    4. kept stationary at the location of the fetal head.

17. Which of these actions should most certainly have been taken by the nurse prior to listening to the fetal heart rate?
    1. Counting the mother's radial pulse.
    2. Ascertaining the height of the uterine fundus.
    3. Determining the station of the fetus.
    4. Palpating the abdomen for fetal position.

18. All of the following are desirable nursing measures for mothers in early labor. Which one did the nurse caring for Maureen carry out?
    1. Telling the mother that she will be able to receive medication for discomfort associated with her contractions.
    2. Encouraging the mother to relax between contractions.
    3. Waiting for the mother's contraction to be over before continuing with a procedure.
    4. Reassuring the mother about the baby's condition.

19. While Maureen was in labor, which of these measures by the nurse would have been desirable in her care?
    1. Offering her oral fluids.
    2. Encouraging her to ambulate.
    3. Coaching her in accelerated breathing techniques.
    4. Asking her if she wanted to listen to the fetal heartbeat.

End of Part 1.
Stop—Do not break the seal until told to do so!

INSTRUCTIONS

Proceed exactly as you did in answering the questions in Part 1 of this test. You will have 15 minutes to take this portion of the test.

20. A judgment that is warranted about the doctor's sitting on Maureen's bed is that it was
    1. unsafe because transmission of disease can occur.
    2. unwise because patients may view such behavior as being unprofessional.
    3. acceptable as a means of establishing a closer relationship with a patient.
    4. permissible on a maternity unit, though it would not be on other hospital units.

21. After the doctor noticed that Maureen's legs were shaking, he told her that the "shaking and shivering would get worse afterwards." Which judgment of the doctor's comment is accurate? (Assume that this is Maureen's first baby.)
    1. Since chills occur less frequently after delivery today than was once true, it was an inappropriate response.
    2. Since multiparas are more susceptible to chills than are primiparas, it was an inappropriate response.
    3. Since emotionally stable patients develop chills more frequently than do emotionally labile ones, it was a premature response.
    4. Since excessive body fluid precipitates chills following delivery, it was a premature response.

22. The doctor's comment to Maureen in question #21 was most likely to
    1. make her more anxious.
    2. alert her to an expectable occurrence.
    3. diminish her confidence in him.
    4. decrease her concern about the shaking.

23. Maureen received intravenous fluids while she was in labor, probably because it was routine practice in that hospital. An accurate understanding, however, of such therapy for women in labor is that it is used
    1. chiefly to prevent fetal dehydration.
    2. primarily to promote the effectiveness of analgesia.
    3. commonly if labor is prolonged.
    4. frequently if the mother's intake of calories was low prior to the onset of labor.

24. At one point in the film when the wall clock in Maureen's room is seen, Maureen says, "The hands never, never, never seemed to move." Which of these understandings about that comment would have been most useful as the basis for responding to Maureen?
    1. Perception of time may be impaired during periods of stress.
    2. Patients who are closely attended by a nurse experience difficulty in assessing time.
    3. The interpretation of time involves symbolism.
    4. Cultural factors tend to affect patients' conceptions of elapsed time.

25. Maureen's apparent conception of the passage of time was evidenced by several comments she made. Which of these comments that the nurse might have made (assuming that the labor was normal) would have been most reassuring?
    1. "Although you are doing satisfactorily, there are no

so-called typical or normal limits."
2. "You are making good steady progress. After a point, it will go more quickly."
3. "Your labor pattern is not unusual. Of course, there is wide variation in the length of labor."
4. "You have been working hard, but labor is hard work."

26. Which of these observations about Maureen's care is *most* justifiable in relation to the giving of medications to her?
1. Personnel failed to give her information about the intended effects of the medications.
2. Measures were not taken by the nurse to allay discomfort between medications.
3. There was a hesitancy on the part of staff to administer any medication.
4. She was made to feel that she would be violating the principles of prepared childbirth if she were to be medicated.

27. At one point when Maureen was very uncomfortable, the doctor told her that he didn't want her to have "too many medicines." Medications are given judiciously at the end of the first stage of labor to prevent which of these conditions?
1. Depression of the infant.
2. Too rapid expulsion of the baby.
3. Uterine atony.
4. Clouding of the mother's sensoria.

28. While the doctor was examining Maureen's rectum, which of these actions by the nurse was especially *UNDESIRABLE* in terms of Maureen's emotional needs?

1. Leaving Maureen's lower abdomen and legs exposed.
2. Standing in back of the doctor rather than next to Maureen.
3. Failing to explain to Maureen what was being done.
4. Neglecting to confer with the doctor promptly about the extent of Maureen's discomfort.

29. While Maureen was being examined by the doctor, the nurse *FAILED* to provide for
1. proper positioning of Maureen for the procedure.
2. disposal of the equipment used by the doctor.
3. adequate draping of Maureen's legs.
4. visibility of the area.

30. When Jean is about to go off duty, she brings in Kathy, the nurse who will take over. After Maureen thanks Jean, she says, "I hope I won't be here when you come back," to which Kathy comments, "Don't worry about that— you won't be."
Which of these judgments about Kathy's response is defensible?
1. Although the first part of the response was nonspecific, the second part was positively stated and therefore would alleviate a patient's anxiety.
2. A response which included the probable duration of labor would have been preferable.
3. Such responses are ineffective in reassuring patients; a more specific response would have been more effective.
4. Patients disregard the actual content of a nurse's response if the manner and tone of the response are pleasant.

31. Maureen's comments during labor should lead one to conclude that she was
    1. unusually anxious.
    2. anticipating a prolonged labor.
    3. eager for the presence of another person.
    4. favorably impressed with the medical and nursing staffs.

32. Which of these approaches by the nurse would have been *most* supportive to Maureen toward the end of the first stage of labor?
    1. Telling her the station of the presenting part.
    2. Telling her that she would soon be able to push.
    3. Telling her that she would soon be able to have an analgesic.
    4. Telling her that her labor was more than half over.

33. Three of the following statements describing the nurses' behavior toward Maureen are justifiable. Which one is *NOT?*
    1. They talked *at* her rather than *with* her.
    2. They never followed through to find out what she was thinking about or needed.
    3. They made assumptions about her based upon other assumptions.
    4. They demonstrated negative feelings toward her.

34. While Maureen was in labor, the nurses giving her care *FAILED* to provide
    1. a quiet environment conducive to rest and relaxation.
    2. instruction in how to work with contractions.
    3. physical comfort measures.
    4. equipment to promote safety.

35. Staff could have contributed to the potential danger of anoxia in Maureen's infant chiefly by
    1. not encouraging Maureen to carry out deep-breathing exercises between contractions.
    2. allowing Maureen to assume the position she found most comfortable.
    3. not offering a bedpan to Maureen.
    4. keeping Maureen flat in bed.

36. The nurse coached Maureen in breathing techniques. Which judgment of the nurse's approach and method is accurate?
    1. The approach was appropriate, and the method was acceptable.
    2. The approach was appropriate, but the method was unacceptable.
    3. The approach was inappropriate, but the method was acceptable.
    4. The approach was inappropriate, and the method was unacceptable.

37. Which of these statements accurately assesses the reaction of personnel to Maureen when she was experiencing discomfort associated with contractions?
    1. The doctor was more responsive to her than were the nurses.
    2. The nurses were more supportive of her than was the doctor.
    3. There was essentially no difference between the behavior of the doctor and the nurses toward her.
    4. The actions of the admitting nurse were more like those of the doctor than were those of the nurse who cared for her later.

End of Part 2.
Stop—Do not break the seal until told to do so!

INSTRUCTIONS
Proceed exactly as you did in answering the questions in Part 2 of this test. You will have 20 minutes to take this portion of the test.

38. The clock in Maureen's room was visible at various times. On the basis of the passage of time gleaned from the film, which of these judgments of the length of Maureen's labor as a primigravida is warranted?
    1. Maureen's labor appeared to fit the normal pattern.
    2. The first stage of Maureen's labor was within normal limits, but the second stage seemed to be prolonged.
    3. The first stage of Maureen's labor was unusually long, but the second stage was within the normal range.
    4. There was insufficient data to allow a conclusion about the duration of Maureen's labor.

39. As the delivery room nurse was scrubbing Maureen's perineum, she said, "I hope you can't feel the solution because it's hot." Maureen did not reply, and the nurse continued with the procedure. Which judgment is relevant in this situation?
    1. Since Maureen is likely to be experiencing loss of sensation in the perineal area following the epidural block, she may be burned by the solution.
    2. Since a temperature above that comfortable for most persons must be used in the delivery room to obtain satisfactory skin disinfection, the nurse's action was appropriate.
    3. Since relief of discomfort associated with strong contractions is promoted when warmed solutions are used topically, the solution would produce a therapeutic effect.
    4. Since hospital practice dictates what temperature should be used for skin preparation solution as well as the type of solution, the nurse was apparently performing correctly.

40. Which aspect of Maureen's management while she was in the delivery room would generally be considered most INEFFECTIVE?
    1. Having her push while lying flat.
    2. Keeping her hands restrained.
    3. Coaching her during contractions without being specific.
    4. Not keeping a hand on her abdomen continuously.

41. On the basis of the information provided in the film, the probable rationale for the use of forceps with Maureen was to
    1. adhere to medical policy.
    2. shorten the second stage of labor.
    3. facilitate delivery of a large baby.
    4. prevent perineal tears.

42. A procedure usually carried out immediately after delivery of the placenta that was NOT seen in the film was
    1. administering an oxytocic.
    2. performing the Credé maneuver.
    3. discontinuing the intravenous infusion.
    4. evaluating the amount of blood loss.

43. Which of these measures was carried out first following the baby's delivery?
    1. Cleansing his face of secretions.
    2. Cutting the umbilical cord.
    3. Suctioning his airway.
    4. Obtaining his Apgar score.

44. Which of the following aspects of the Apgar scoring system was performed by the nurse in the delivery room?
    1. Evaluating the infant's color.
    2. Evaluating the infant's muscle tone.
    3. Counting the infant's respirations.
    4. Counting the infant's apical heart rate.

45. The one aspect of the baby's management in the delivery room that could most justifiably be criticized was that he was
    1. not given to his mother soon enough.
    2. held by the doctor with only one hand.
    3. placed on his mother's abdomen prior to delivery of the placenta.
    4. examined rather superficially for congenital anomalies.

46. While Maureen was in the delivery room, she was given her baby to hold. Which behavior demonstrated by Maureen is the most significant part of the maternal "claiming" process, according to Rubin?
    1. Extending her arms to receive him.
    2. Cuddling him.
    3. Trying to establish eye contact with him while talking to him.
    4. Using her fingers to explore his face.

47. Which of these measures should most certainly be carried out before the baby is transferred to the nursery?
    1. Cleansing him of blood and vernix caseosa.
    2. Applying an identification device to him.
    3. Covering his umbilical stump with a sterile dressing.
    4. Taking his vital signs.

48. At the end of the film, when Maureen commented, "The baby was inside me for nine months and now here he is," the doctor answered, "You did a good job." Which of these assessments of his comment is justifiable?
    1. It was made before the patient's remark was clarified.
    2. It immediately reinforced positive behavior in the patient.
    3. It was a complimentary acknowledgement of the patient's reaction.
    4. It reinforced the reality of the baby's arrival for the patient.

49. During the first hour after Maureen's delivery, which of these measures will be essential in her care?
    1. Taking her vital signs every 10 minutes.
    2. Giving her perineal care.
    3. Evaluating the tone of her uterine fundus.
    4. Changing her gown after bathing her.

50. At various points in the film, personnel tried to reassure Maureen by giving her pat statements. The chief DISADVANTAGE of such reponses is that they
    1. reduce the patient's confidence in the competence of staff.
    2. tend to close off communication.
    3. are not focused on patient needs.
    4. relay only superficial information.

51. Which of these interpretations is most justifiable about the nurse-doctor relationship in the film?
   1. There appeared to be an interaction commonly called "professional" between them.
   2. There seemed to be a feeling of mutual respect between them.
   3. There was little or no communication between them.
   4. There did not seem to be any independent action on the part of doctors or nurses in relation to the patient's management.

52. Which of these generalizations should a nurse have about the effect of doctor-nurse relationships on patients like Maureen in a situation such as the one depicted in the film?
   1. If any disagreement between doctors and nurses is perceived by the patient, it might be interpreted by the patient as a potential threat to her.
   2. Patients in labor are so self-centered that they are unaware of doctors' and nurses' behaviors.
   3. An attitude of joviality and lightheartedness on the part of doctors and nurses contributes to an anxiety-free experience for the patient.
   4. The behavior of doctors and nurses as individuals is more important than the relationships between and among them.

53. From both verbal and non-verbal interactions between Maureen and the nurses, it is reasonable to infer that
   1. there was a lack of affective feelings evident in their relationships with Maureen.
   2. the nurses' behavior toward Maureen is typical of the way most nurses treat maternity patients regardless of their marital status.
   3. the calmness exhibited by the nurses is synonymous with acceptance of Maureen as a person.
   4. there was an absence of judgment on the part of Maureen and the nurses.

54. The film does not tell whether Maureen has had a baby previously or whether she has ever seen a delivery. If personnel had had such information, it would have been *most* useful as the
   1. basis for teaching, since knowing where the patient "is" allows the nurse to be more helpful.
   2. means by which the nurse could review and reiterate pertinent information.
   3. frame of reference for establishing a nursing care plan.
   4. mechanism by which a meaningful nurse-patient relationship could be established.

55. Since Maureen made no mention of preparation for the baby's care, it would be safest to apply which of the following understandings?
   1. There is a direct relationship between the amount of preparation a woman makes for her baby and her financial resources.
   2. The preparation that a pregnant woman makes for her baby is directly related to the size of the family she anticipates having.
   3. Cultural factors influence significantly the extent to which a woman prepares for her baby during pregnancy.
   4. Rejection of the pregnancy by a woman interferes with her preparing for her baby's arrival.

56. An assumption seemed to be made by personnel about Maureen and her baby. This assumption was that Maureen
    1. was disappointed in the baby's sex.
    2. needed help in coming to a decision about the baby's future.
    3. was uncertain about her ability to take care of the baby.
    4. planned to keep the baby.

57. The most obvious *OMISSION* in the film was any reference to Maureen's
    1. feelings about giving birth.
    2. relationship with the baby's father.
    3. decision about the feeding of her baby.
    4. general health status.

58. The segment of the film that correctly demonstrates aseptic technique involved the
    1. shaving of the perineum prior to delivery.
    2. administration of the enema prior to delivery.
    3. wearing of masks in the delivery room.
    4. preparation of the perineum in the delivery room.

59. If a group of primigravidas were to view the film, what general effect might be expected?
    1. Anxiety, because many points about labor and delivery were not covered.
    2. Satisfaction of curiosity, because some aspects of having a baby were made evident.
    3. Disappointment, because only the mother's role was shown.
    4. Disillusionment, because the joy of childbearing was not made explicit while the pain was.

60. If the film were to be shown to a group of pregnant women, it would be desirable to include all of the following measures in the program. Which one would it be essential to include?
    1. Taking them on a tour of the local obstetric facilities.
    2. Giving them demonstrations of some of the procedures shown in the film.
    3. Holding pre- and post-discussions with them.
    4. Arranging for their husbands to see the film.

This is the end of the test.
Please make certain that you have answered all of the questions and erased any stray marks that you may have made on your answer sheet.

REFERENCES

1. American Psychological Association. *Standards for Educational and Psychological Tests and Manuals.* Washington, D.C.: American Psychological Assoc., 1974.
2. Anastasi, A. *Psychological Testing* (2nd ed.). New York: Macmillan, 1961. Pp. 148–149.
3. *Birth Day – Through the Eyes of the Mother* (film) (Lawrence A. Williams, Producer.) Burlingame, Calif.: Lawren Productions, Inc., 1970.
4. Bloom, B. S. (Ed.). *Taxonomy of Educational Objectives. Handbook I: Cognitive Domain.* New York: David McKay, 1956. Pp. 201–207.
5. Bormuth, J. R. *On the Theory of Achievement Test Items.* Chicago: University of Chicago Press, 1970. Pp. 11–77.
6. Briggs, L., Campeau, P., Gagne, R., and May, M. *Instructional Media: A Procedure for the Design of Multi-Media Instruction, A Critical Review of Research, and Suggestions for Future Research.* Pittsburgh, Pa.: American Institutes for Research, 1967. P. 115.
7. Cronbach, L. J. Course improvement through evaluation. *Teach. Coll. Rec.* 54: 681, 1963.
8. Cronbach, L. J. Test Validation. In R. L. Thorndike (Ed.), *Educational Measurement* (2nd ed.). Washington, D.C.: American Council on Education, 1971. P. 444.
9. Croxton, F. E., Cowden, D. J., and Klein, S. *Applied General Statistics* (3rd ed.). Englewood Cliffs, N. J.: Prentice-Hall, 1967. P. 204.
10. Curtis, H. A., and Kropp, R. P. *Experimental Analyses of the Effects of Various Modes of Item Presentation on the Scores and Factorial Content of Tests Administered by Visual and Audio-Visual Means: A Program of Studies Basic to Television Testing.* Tallahassee, Fla.: Florida State University, n.d. Pp. 13, 77, 82.
11. Gronlund, N. E. *Stating Behavioral Objectives for Classroom Instruction.* New York: Macmillan, 1970. P. 21.
12. Guilford, J. P., and Fruchter, B. *Fundamental Statistics in Psychology and Education* (5th ed.). New York: McGraw-Hill, 1973. Pp. 158–159, 416, 418–419.
13. Henrysson, S. Gathering, Analyzing, and Using Data on Test Items. In R. L. Thorndike (Ed.), *Educational Measurement* (2nd ed.). Washington, D.C.: American Council on Education, 1971. P. 152.
14. Kropp, R. P., and Stoker, H. W. *The Construction and Validation of Tests of the Cognitive Processes as Described in the Taxonomy of Educational Objectives.* Tallahassee, Fla.: Florida State University Institute of Human Learning and Department of Educational Research and Testing, 1966. Pp. 21, 48.
15. Lord, F. M., and Novick, M. R. *Statistical Theories of Mental Test Scores.* Reading, Mass.: Addison-Wesley, 1968. P. 329.
16. Magnusson, D. *Test Theory.* Reading, Mass.: Addison-Wesley, 1966. P. 118.
17. Mandrillo, M. P. A Comparative Study of Cognitive Skills of the Graduating Baccalaureate Degree and Associate Degree Nursing Students. Ed.D. dissertation, Teachers College, Columbia University, 1969. P. 50.
18. National League for Nursing. Let's examine—reliability. *Nurs. Outlook* 19:120, 1971.
19. *National Survey of Audiovisual Materials for Nursing – 1968-1969* (Conducted by the ANA-NLN Film Service). New York: The American Journal of Nursing Company, Educational Services Division, 1970.
20. Seibert, W. F., Snow, R. E., and Senn, J. E. Jr. *Studies in Cine-Psychometry 1: Preliminary Factor Analysis of Visual Cognition and*

Memory. Lafayette, Ind.: Purdue University Audio-Visual Center, 1965. Pp. 2, 16-22.

21. Stanley, J. C. and Hopkins, K. D.   *Education and Psychological Measurement and Evaluation.* Englewood Cliffs, N.J.: Prentice-Hall, 1972. Pp. 101–102.

22. Thorndike, R. L.   *Personnel Selection.* New York: Wiley & Sons, 1949. P. 42.

23. Thorndike, R. L., and Hagen, E.   *Measurement and Evaluation in Psychology and Education* (4th ed.). New York: Wiley & Sons, 1977. Pp. 49–50, 215, 250.

24. Tinkelman, S. N.   Planning the Objective Test. In R.L. Thorndike (Ed.), *Educational Measurement* (2nd ed.). Washington, D.C.: American Council on Education, 1971. Pp. 63–64.

SUGGESTED READING FOR FILM-MAKING

1. Bobker, L. R.   *Elements of Film.* New York: Harcourt, Brace & World, 1969.

2. Cushman, G.   *Movie Making in 18 Lessons.* New York: E. P. Dutton, 1971.

3. Eastman Kodak Co.   *How to Make Good Sound Movies.* Rochester, N.Y.: Eastman Kodak, 1973.

4. Ferguson, R.   *How to Make Movies.* New *York:* Viking Press, 1969.

5. Goldstein, L. and Kaufman, J.   *Into Film.* New York:E. P. Dutton, 1976.

6. Linder, C. *Filmmaking—A Practical Guide.* Englewood Cliffs, N.J.: Prentice-Hall, 1976.

7. Lipton, L.   *Independent Film Making.* San Francisco: Straight Arrow Books, 1972.

8. Lipton, L.   *The Super 8 Book.* San Francisco: Straight Arrow Books, 1975.

9. Matzkin, M. A.   *Super 8 mm Movie Making Simplified.* New York: Amphoto, 1975.

10. Pincus, E.   *Guide to Filmmaking.* New York: New American Library, 1972.

11. Rose T.   *The Complete Book of Movie Making.* New York: Morgan & Morgan, 1971.

12. Smallman, K.   *Creative Film-Making.* New York: Bantam Books, 1972.

13. Wallace, C.   *Making Movies.* London: Evans Brothers Ltd., 1965.

14. Yulsman, J.   *The Complete Book of 8 mm Movie Making.* New York: Barnes & Noble, 1972.

4. Evaluation of Clinical Performance by Direct Observation

Paper-and-pencil tests can very accurately measure what a nurse knows. They can, and often do, ask what a nurse would do in a particular situation and the nurse could answer the question correctly; in other words, a written test assesses the cognitive aspects of clinical performance. But, what the nurse would actually do in a real situation can only be determined by observing how the nurse performs in that situation. A common example of tests that assess the cognitive aspects of nursing performance are the State Board Test Pool Examinations for nurse licensure. In addition to questions on facts and principles relevant to the purpose of the examination—safety and effectiveness of nursing practice—and the application of those facts and principles, a large proportion of the questions are geared to the cognitive components of clinical nursing practice: what *should* the nurse do? Faculty in some schools of nursing seem surprised when told that since the licensing examination measures only cognitive aspects, it is essential that *they*, the faculty, "certify" the ability of their nursing students to perform competently in the clinical setting and thus be ready to sit for the licensing examination. It would seem by this attitude that they wanted the licensing examination, not themselves, to weed out the incompetent from the competent nurse practitioner in terms of their ability to *give* nursing care.

Observation of the nurse in the process of giving nursing care can be accomplished in a number of ways, for example, randomly—by nurse, by patient, by setting, by time—or on a scheduled, systematic basis. It can be done without the benefit of aids, or some kind of guidelines can be used. Haphazard observations without detailing specifically what is to be observed are useless and meaningless, as well as costly in terms of observers' time.

When the content of clinical performance tools in use in some schools of nursing is compared with the appropriate course objectives, one would question the derivation of the clinical performance objectives from curriculum objectives, and specifically in relation to course objectives. The two sets of objectives appear completely unrelated to each other. Unfortunately, evaluation and the necessary tools for evaluation seem to be relegated to the last phase of course development. It is a recognized need but since the job is so difficult, it is only appended to the course package. If faculty only realized how much easier it would be to consider evaluation procedures concurrently with subject-matter objectives, the development of behavioral objectives would be viewed with an eye to their observability and therefore their measurability.

A problem frequently seen in clinical performance evaluation tools is the inappropriateness of some of the objectives in light of the purpose of the tool, that is, to evaluate the nurse's ability to *perform.* If cognitive objectives were eliminated (to the degree possible) from clinical performance evaluation tools, and if only psychomotor objectives were included, the instructor could focus on the nurse's performance. The result would be more meaningful and valid, and would provide useful information about the student's ability to perform. An objective such as "Identifies and interprets abnormal diagnostic data" can be more efficiently and reliably measured in a paper-and-pencil test. In addition, that objective really consists of two parts and is therefore inappropriate for the purpose of measurement. The student may be able to identify abnormal diagnostic data but be unable to interpret that data. How then could attainment of that objective be recorded? Another example of a cognitive objective inappropriate for a performance tool is "Understands the legal implications of nursing actions." With a little ingenuity, a number of test questions could be developed to assess that objective quite accurately. I am not advocating the elimination of all cognitive objectives from clinical performance evaluation tools, only that faculty be aware that direct observation of clinical performance should be confined to that which is overtly observable. Some faculty members have reacted strongly to the suggestion that they eliminate as many of the cognitive objectives as possible. However, many of these types of objectives that they are concerned about can be assessed during pre- and postconferences, by oral questioning, or in short written quizzes and thus will not be overlooked.

A nurse may place a newly admitted patient with leukemia into protective or reverse isolation but this action cannot be interpreted to mean that the nurse "Interprets abnormal diagnostic data," or "Understands the implications of low white blood cell counts in patients with leukemia," or "Identifies the need for patients with leukemia to be protected from infection." The nurse may have placed the patient in protective isolation *solely* because the physician wrote an order to do just that. We cannot assume—at least not without supporting data—that when a nurse takes a specific action, it is because she understands the underlying basis, the rationale, for that action (although it would make the process of evaluation a lot easier). Some novice faculty members find it difficult to accept that this is so, however.

Another common problem with behavioral objectives pertains to their lack of specificity. Some objectives listed on clinical performance evaluation tools are so global that one of them could cover an entire course. Take the objective "Uses the nursing process in the care of patients." Suppose that a nursing student did (1) a fantastic job of assessing a patient's needs, (2) a fairly good job in planning for his needs, (3) satisfactorily implemented the plan, and (4) was unable to evaluate the outcomes of the plan. How could the student's attainment of that four-part objective possibly be assessed?

Objectives, particularly clinical performance objectives, need to be broken down into elements that are discrete and independently measurable. This process may result in a long list of behavioral objectives that may overwhelm faculty and students alike in terms of achievement and evaluation but it is a necessary step. What should then be done is to check the list for duplication or overlapping, or both. A fairly common reaction of faculty to the discrete behavioral objectives is that because they are so specific, they may appear to be task- or procedure-oriented and therefore inapplicable to a program that purports to teach a "high level" of nursing practice.

PRINCIPLES OF EVALUATION AS RELATED TO OBSERVATION

Mention must be made of two maxims of evaluation that are not universally adhered to and are not mutually exclusive. First, trite as it may sound, students must have the opportunity to learn before they are evaluated. Secondly, the purpose of evaluating the nursing student's performance needs to be identified. Is the reason for evaluating the performance chiefly to help the student master the task or material (formative evaluation) or is it for the purpose of assigning a grade or a rating (summative evaluation)?

One of the principles of effective evaluation is to use guidelines to direct the observation of performance. Such guidelines can be couched either in general terms or in simple statements about the expected behavior in a satisfactory nursing performance at the appropriate level. Better still, examples of nursing behaviors can be given for above average, average, and below average abilities. Gradations beyond these three are difficult to specify but can and have been done.

Rating scales and checklists are especially helpful in directing observations, if these tools contain the discrete, observable behaviors previously mentioned. Much too often the focus is on personality traits rather than behaviors, which can create another problem. If personality traits are being assessed (and probably not very well), the person being evaluated is likely to have a strongly negative reaction to the process since he may feel he is being personally attacked. In contrast, if evaluation is focused on behavioral traits, it is the performance being critiqued, not the performer.

Although the majority of faculty members give students necessary written materials early in the course, for example, the course objectives, the bibliography, and the criteria for written assignments, not all of them give the students the clinical performance evaluation tools, either at the outset of the course or before they are evaluated. And there really is no reason why students shouldn't know the method and criteria by which they will be evaluated. Additionally, since self-evaluation is advocated, what better way to accomplish this than to have students evaluate themselves as they progress in the course, using the same tool as the instructor, and not just prior to graduation.

It would also be desirable for the tool to have the same format for each course in the curriculum. Obviously each course has unique objectives in addition to those that progress through the curriculum, and these should be reflected in the tool, but the same format will ease the student's adaptation and acceptance of the tool. The process of evaluation is stressful and can be grueling enough for the student without the extra and unnecessary burden of adjusting to a tool with a different format in each course.

Some faculty members are uncomfortable when using a checklist or rating scale, in part because the task seems so easy; they feel the need to write "volumes" of notes, that is, anecdotal notes, regarding a student's performance. Too, an increasing number of legal entanglements in recent years brought about by former students (and former employees) has caused an accompanying concern for adequate documentation of a person's performance. The problem with the use of anecdotal notes is that although they have been kept on students from the first day they are assigned to a unit until the day they leave, the notes are *summarized* into a final evaluation. This practice violates one of the principles of evaluation in terms of assigning a grade or a rank—students have been evaluated while they are learning! When anecdotal notes accompany a checklist or rating scale that has been used at a specific time on a particular day, the anecdotes *must* pertain to that time frame. What to include in such a note is a question frequently raised. Two examples may be useful and are illustrated below. Note that the instructor's comments and judgments are separated from the recording of the incident.

Samples of Anecdotal Notes

Student B. J. Jones   *Place* Newborn Nursery   *Date* 5/30/77
                                                   Observer H. Shore
Miss Jones was caring for a 3-day-old normal newborn. Infant had loose, sticky transitional stool. Student wiped off stool from buttocks with clean corner of diaper, put diaper next to infant's head, and then attempted to remove remaining stool from buttocks with dry cotton, causing skin to become quite reddened. Discarded diaper and proceeded with remaining care and inspection without washing her hands.

(Student was reminded yesterday to wash hands before going from an infant's unit to a "clean" area.)

Student S. Smith   *Place* Toddlers' Unit   *Date* 4/30/77
                                                   Observer H. Shore
Miss Smith was assigned to care for 18-month-old with LTB who was in Croupette. Doctor's order reads: "Try out of Croupette." Child's mother at bedside. Child crying, reaching out to mother as if wanting to be picked up. Student asks mother to please wait in parents' waiting room until child's care is completed, at which time the mother would be notified and then may return.

(Miss Smith has on several occasions seemed to be uncomfortable in the presence of parents. In conferences verbalizes need of children for their parents, especially during stressful situations.)

One of the practices that deserves serious consideration is the scheduling of performance tests just as paper-and-pencil tests are scheduled, an approach used by Peterson and colleagues [29]. There undoubtedly will be problems associated with this technique, e.g., the logistical one: juggling the number of students to be tested with the number of instructors available to assist with the testing. Another problem would be the sampling of content to be included in the test. With a paper-and-pencil test, a blueprint of specifications immensely aids the sampling process, and perhaps the same kind of approach would facilitate sampling from the performance aspects of nursing. What might be tried in conjunction with the blueprint, or perhaps separately, is randomly assigning students to different nursing care situations. Student A might be assigned to the care of a child in a Croupette, while Student B could be assigned to the care of an infant with diarrhea, and so on. While some of these aspects of direct patient care could be tested in a simulated laboratory (see Chap. 7), others can only be tested in the real situation.

DEVELOPING AN EVALUATION TOOL

When faced with the task of creating a tool to be used for evaluating the ability of nurses to perform, a frequently heard question is "Where do we begin?" Clinical performance objectives derive from course objectives and can be identified in part by the behaviors contained therein. Verbs such as "palpates," "administers," "teaches," "interviews," and "maintains" describe the kinds of behaviors that can probably be assessed only by direct observation. One way to determine which objectives are cognitive, which ones affective, and which ones psychomotor has been shown in Table 3-1. It should be reiterated here, however, that some objectives can be tested both cognitively and behaviorally, for example, those in the "adapts" category. See also the work of Peterson and associates [29] for some objectives that are in the cognitive domain but are directly related to clinical performance.

A decision that should be made early is how clinical performance will be graded or rated. Will a system of pass/fail; satisfactory/unsatisfactory; above average, average, and below average be used; or will a grade of A, B, C, etc., or the equivalent numbers be used? When that is decided, criteria will need to be written to indicate what constitutes satisfactory performance, what unsatisfactory performance, and the like. Such criteria are essential, particularly when a system of grades used. What differentiates an A student from a B student, or a C student from a D or F student? This specific differentiation is what is lacking in many performance tools in schools that use letter grades or their numerical equivalents. A related consideration pertains to how clinical performance grades will be treated in relation to theory grades. In some schools satisfactory performance in the clinical part of the course is mandatory in order to pass the course. (This practice reflects my own philosophy since nursing is a "doing" as well as a "knowing" profession.) In other schools, clinical grades count 50% of the course grade, but this practice is unjustifiable unless a clear distinction has been made between the A, B, C, etc., clinical performance grades previously mentioned. When theory grades are averaged with clinical grades, it's much like averaging a fresh apple with a hamburger with all the trimmings! Of course, school policy may dictate what can and cannot be done with grades; in these situations a faculty will have to make the effort to change policies incongruent with their identified needs.

Once the clinical performance objectives have been isolated, a next step is to decide the format the tool should take. Whether an evaluation committee or the total faculty is responsible for the decision is not as important as the fact that there should be agreement on the ultimate form. Discussion may focus on "But what if we don't like it or it's hard to use?" The answer should be that if the initial form is found to be deficient in some way, it can be revised later, based on its experimental use. Revision of the form *should* be anticipated, and perhaps more than once.

Concurrent with the decision on format should be the perusal of already available forms, one's own tools as well as those from other schools, and those that have already been published. Several of them may offer possibilities; adapt what is good from any particular form. Of course, the objectives will need to be unique for the individual school and course.

The scoring of checklists and rating scales presents a not-easily-solved problem. One approach is for faculty to decide that all students must satisfactorily perform all of the previously established *critical* elements of nursing care. What constitutes these critical elements, however, may involve countless hours of discussion, with some faculty members never agreeing. The "nice to know" elements are less likely to pose problems. Although the final decision as to the critical elements of a specific course should probably rest with the faculty responsible for the course, the decision to use the critical components approach should be made by the total faculty. In some schools an evaluation committee is charged with such responsibilities. An example of the critical elements approach has been used in the performance examinations of the New York Regents External Degree Program in nursing [20].

Another approach to scoring a checklist or rating scale is suggested by Thorndike and Hagen [36]. In their method, a favorable attribute is given a score of +1, an unfavorable attribute is given a score of -1, and a neutral attribute is given a score of 0. The resulting score would then be a sum of these numbers. How the numbers (the total score) would then be treated is again a decision that faculty will need to make, preferably beforehand and then revised if necessary. Still another method is discussed later in this chapter (see p. 71).

Included in the references are a number of published reports about the development of performance tools. Recent articles include those by Burke and Goodale [3], Haar and Hicks [11], and Nichols and Heydman [26]. Some of the older ones included are worthy of citation because of their comprehensiveness, for example, the works of Dyer [7, 8], Wandelt and Stewart [40], and Tate [33–35].

Criterion Behaviors Checklist

The checklist that will now be described was developed, as was the film test discussed in Chapter 3, for use in evaluating the clinical competence of a geographic sample of baccalaureate nursing students in a unit of obstetric nursing.

DESIGN OF THE CHECKLIST

Since clinical competence involves "doing" as well as "knowing," and since some of the objectives of the labor and delivery unit can only be evaluated by direct observation, a list of criterion behaviors was developed from the previously identified objectives (see pp. 22–24). A distinction between criterion behaviors and critical behaviors should be made clear. The performance of a *criterion* behavior is desirable rather than mandatory, whereas performance of a *critical* behavior is absolutely essential for safe and effective nursing practice. A behavior such as "Fails to teach the patient self-perineal care" might be classified as an unacceptable *criterion* behavior, but "Does not massage a boggy uterine fundus" would undoubtedly be classified by most maternity nurses as an unacceptable *critical* behavior, since hemorrhage and death might result from its omission.

One reason for including criterion behaviors in the checklist is that they would be more representative of what nurses actually do in their care of patients. Although critical behaviors are not likely to occur with any regularity nor with the same frequency as criterion behaviors, thus making assessment impossible for most students, they should be included in case they can be observed. Another important reason why observations should not be limited solely to the critical behaviors is my belief that only the faculty in each school should decide which behaviors *they* deem critical based upon *their* philosophy, educational program, and setting. For these reasons, there is no differentiation made in the list between criterion and critical behaviors and both are included under the single heading "criterion behaviors."

It must be recognized that the criticisms levelled against all such checklists are applicable to this one as well. However, for the purpose for which this tool was designed, the use of the same checklist by all of the instructors in the study schools at least eliminated one common source of error variance (i.e., each school using a different checklist). In addition, the behaviors in the checklist were derived from the unit objectives, were worded so that no judgment needed to be made save whether they (1) were or were not performed, (2) were independently observable, and (3) were felt to be expected and typical behaviors of baccalaureate nursing students following completion of the unit of instruction in normal labor and delivery, and therefore universally applicable. The first version of the checklist that finally evolved follows (see p. 66).

ADMINISTRATION OF THE CHECKLIST

The instructors of the students in the sample were asked to evaluate their students using the checklist. The instructions accompanying the checklist directed the instructor to check the appropriate behavior as being either Acceptable or Unacceptable. The checklist was designed to be used for evaluating a student's performance during a specific time period in one day, and, of course, after the student had had the opportunity to

**Labor and Delivery Clinical Laboratory
Experience: Criterion Behaviors**

Student _____ Date of Observation _____
                                   Observer _____

Directions for Use: Place a ✔ mark next to the behavior observed.
When the period of observation is ended, place a 0 next to any
pair of behaviors for which neither the Acceptable nor the Unacceptable was checked.

Acceptable Behaviors		Unacceptable Behaviors	
1. Introduces self to patient by name and title	☐	Does not introduce self to patient by name and/or title	☐
2. Explains to patient how nurse will participate in her care	☐	Does not explain to patient how nurse will participate in her care	☐
3. Checks patient's valuables and deals with them according to hospital policy	☐	Does not check patient's valuables and deal with them according to hospital policy	☐
4. Wears only a smooth-strapped watch with a second hand	☐	Does not wear a smooth-strapped watch with a second hand and/or wears ring(s) likely to be injurious to patient	☐
5. Uses language appropriate for patient's intellectual level and emotional state when giving instructions or explanations	☐	Does not use language appropriate for patient's intellectual level and/or emotional state when giving instructions or explanations	☐
6. Relates pertinent observations and findings promptly to the instructor	☐	Does not relate pertinent observations and findings promptly to the instructor	☐
7. Records observations and findings accurately and promptly	☐	Does not record observations and findings accurately and promptly	☐
8. Elicits relevant history including symptoms of true labor	☐	Does not elicit relevant history including symptoms of true labor	☐
9. Finds out what patient knows about the process of labor and delivery	☐	Does not find out what patient knows about the process of labor and delivery	☐
10. Palpates patient's abdomen for fetal position before auscultation of the fetal heartbeat	☐	Does not palpate patient's abdomen for fetal position before auscultation of the fetal heartbeat	☐
11. Places fingers on patient's radial artery while listening to the fetal heartbeat for the first time	☐	Does not place fingers on patient's radial artery while listening to the fetal heartbeat for the first time	☐
12. Takes fetal heart rate after contractions, after rupture of the membranes, and after the administration of medications	☐	Does not take fetal heart rate after contractions, after rupture of the membranes, and after the administration of medications	☐
13. Takes patient's vital signs	☐	Does not take patient's vital	☐

Acceptable Behaviors		Unacceptable Behaviors	
following the administration of medications and/or anesthesia and at appropriate intervals otherwise		signs following the administration of medications and/or anesthesia and at appropriate intervals otherwise	
14. Times uterine contractions accurately and at appropriate intervals	☐	Does not time uterine contractions accurately and at appropriate intervals	☐
15. Explains purpose and procedure of the perineal preparation and enema before proceeding with the procedure	☐	Does not explain purpose and procedure of the perineal preparation and enema before proceeding with the procedure	☐
16. Performs the admission procedures correctly, e.g., perineal shave, enema, urine specimen	☐	Does not perform the admission procedures correctly, e.g., perineal shave, enema, urine specimen	☐
17. Permits patient to ambulate until her membranes rupture, according to hospital policy	☐	Does not permit patient to ambulate until her membranes rupture, according to hospital policy	☐
18. Encourages patient to breathe abdominally, deeply, and slowly during contractions in the early first stage of labor	☐	Does not encourage patient to breathe abdominally, deeply, and slowly during contractions in the early first stage of labor	☐
19. Encourages patient to relax between contractions	☐	Does not encourage patient to relax between contractions	☐
20. Permits patient to express herself freely without interjection of inappropriate comments	☐	Does not permit patient to express herself freely without interjection of inappropriate comments	☐
21. Alleviates patient's fears and reduces her tension to the degree possible by using various appropriate means	☐	Does not alleviate patient's fears nor reduce her tension to the degree possible by using various appropriate means	☐
22. Keeps patient and her husband apprised of the progress of labor	☐	Does not keep patient and her husband apprised of the progress of labor	☐
23. Encourages husband to participate in his wife's care	☐	Does not encourage husband to participate in his wife's care	☐
24. Encourages patient to pant during contractions at the end of the first stage of labor	☐	Does not encourage patient to pant during contractions at the end of the first stage of labor	☐
25. Institutes nursing measures to promote patient comfort, such as back rubs, mouth rinses, sponge baths, perineal care	☐	Does not institute nursing measures to promote patient comfort, such as back rubs, mouth rinses, sponge baths, perineal care	☐
26. Administers oral fluids according to hospital policy	☐	Does not administer oral fluids according to hospital policy	☐
27. Interprets the purpose of intravenous fluids when they are instituted, and carries out the same routine with the maternity patient	☐	Does not interpret the purpose of intravenous fluids when they are instituted, nor carry out the same routine with the maternity patient as with	☐

Acceptable Behaviors		Unacceptable Behaviors	
as with other adult patients		other adult patients	
28. Assists patient with positioning to facilitate respiratory exchange, pushing efforts, and the administration of anesthetics, and to prevent postural hypotension	☐	Does not assist patient with positioning to facilitate respiratory exchange, pushing efforts, and the administration of anesthetics, and to prevent postural hypotension	☐
29. Prepares and administers medications accurately	☐	Does not prepare and administer medications accurately	☐
30. Interprets to the patient the procedure to be used to anesthetize her	☐	Does not interpret to the patient the procedure to be used to anesthetize her	☐
31. Puts side rails up after patient has been medicated or has received an anesthetic agent	☐	Does not put side rails up after patient has been medicated or has received an anesthetic agent	☐
32. Observes perineum for bulging and crowning	☐	Does not observe perineum for bulging and crowning	☐
33. Completely covers nose and mouth with mask when the perineum is exposed in the labor room and during delivery	☐	Does not completely cover nose and mask when the perineum is exposed in the labor room and/or during delivery	☐
34. Removes mask when it is not needed and changes it when it becomes moist	☐	Does not remove mask when it is not needed nor change it when it becomes moist	☐
35. Checks the delivery room to be sure that it has all necessary equipment in readiness—sterile instruments, basins, linen, and a heated crib with resuscitation equipment	☐	Does not check the delivery room to be sure that it has all necessary equipment in readiness—sterile instruments, basins, linen, and heated crib with resuscitation equipment	☐
36. Encourages patient to void at periodic intervals and before being taken to the delivery room	☐	Does not encourage patient to void at periodic intervals nor before being taken to the delivery room	☐
37. Transfers patient from bed to stretcher and vice versa safely	☐	Does not transfer patient from bed to stretcher and vice versa safely	☐
38. Completely covers hair with scrub cap in the delivery room	☐	Does not completely cover hair with scrub cap in the delivery room	☐
39. Places patient in lithotomy position on the delivery table, putting both legs in stirrups at the same time	☐	Does not place patient in lithotomy position on the delivery table, putting both legs in stirrups at the same time	☐
40. Restrains patient's hands if indicated	☐	Does not restrain patient's hands if indicated	☐
41. Checks fetal heart rate at least every 5 minutes	☐	Does not check fetal heart rate at least every 5 minutes	☐
42. Encourages patient to push with each contraction	☐	Does not encourage patient to push with each contraction	☐
43. Cleanses perineum according	☐	Does not cleanse perineum	☐

Acceptable Behaviors		Unacceptable Behaviors	
to hospital policy, using aseptic technique		according to hospital policy, using aseptic technique	
44. Accurately administers medications, e.g., oxytocics, during delivery or after delivery of the placenta depending on hospital policy	☐	Does not accurately administer medication, e.g., oxytocics, during delivery or after delivery of the placenta depending on hospital policy	☐
45. Disposes of placenta according to hospital policy	☐	Does not dispose of placenta according to hospital policy	☐
46. Records observations and other required information accurately and promptly, e.g., Apgar score and time of delivery of infant and of placenta	☐	Does not record observations and other required information accurately and promptly, e.g., Apgar score and time of delivery of infant and of placenta	☐
47. Conducts an infant appraisal using the Apgar scoring system at one minute and five minutes after birth	☐	Does not conduct an infant appraisal using the Apgar scoring system at one minute and five minutes after birth or does it (them) inaccurately	☐
48. Notifies instructor of an Apgar score below 7	☐	Does not notify instructor of an Apgar score below 7	☐
49. Performs those procedures dictated by hospital policy for newborns, e.g., weighing, temperature by rectum, instillation of eye medication, identification of baby and mother, administration of vitamin K	☐	Does not perform those procedures dictated by hospital policy for newborns, e.g., weighing, temperature by rectum, instillation of eye medication, identification of baby and mother, and administration of vitamin K, or performs it (them) inaccurately	☐
50. Keeps infant warm	☐	Does not keep infant warm	☐
51. Appraises infant quickly for gross anomalies	☐	Does not appraise infant quickly for gross anomalies	☐
52. Keeps infant positioned to maintain patency of the airway with drainage of mucus	☐	Does not keep infant positioned to maintain patency of the airway with drainage of mucus	☐
53. Shows infant to his mother after wiping blood and secretions off head	☐	Does not show infant to his mother nor wipe blood and secretions off head	☐
54. Gives breast care before mother breast-feeds her infant	☐	Does not give breast care before mother breast-feeds her infant	☐
55. Assists the breast-feeding mother in helping her infant to nurse	☐	Does not assist the breast-feeding mother in helping her infant to nurse or assists incorrectly	☐
56. Checks infant's identification with the mother before the baby is transferred to the nursery	☐	Does not check infant's identification with the mother before baby is transferred to the nursery	☐
57. Transfers infant to the nursery according to hospital policy	☐	Does not transfer infant to the nursery according to hospital policy	☐

Acceptable Behaviors		Unacceptable Behaviors	
58. Removes patient's legs from the stirrups at the same time	☐	Does not remove patient's legs from the stirrups at the same time	☐
59. Applies perineal pad; examines it and the pad under patient every 15 minutes for amount of lochia	☐	Does not apply perineal pad; does not examine it and the pad under patient every 15 minutes for amount of lochia	☐
60. Notifies instructor if lochia is excessive	☐	Does not notify instructor if lochia is excessive	☐
61. Keeps a hand on the uterine fundus for the first hour after delivery	☐	Does not keep a hand on the uterine fundus for the first hour after delivery	☐
62. Massages uterine fundus correctly if boggy	☐	Does not massage uterine fundus correctly if boggy	☐
63. Notifies instructor if uterine fundus is boggy	☐	Does not notify instructor if uterine fundus is boggy	☐
64. Takes vital signs at specified intervals	☐	Does not take vital signs at specified intervals	☐
65. Encourages patient to void, noting amount	☐	Does not encourage patient to void, noting amount	☐
66. Gives perineal care after patient uses the bedpan for the first time postpartum	☐	Does not give perineal care after patient uses the bedpan for the first time postpartum	☐
67. Bathes patient after delivery, partially or completely, as warranted	☐	Does not bathe patient after delivery, partially or completely, as warranted	☐
68. Changes gown and bed linens as necessary	☐	Does not change gown and bed linens as necessary	☐
69. Examines the episiotomy for oozing and hematomas	☐	Does not examine the episiotomy for oozing and hematomas	☐
70. Arranges for the new family to be together as soon as possible after delivery	☐	Does not arrange for the new family to be together as soon as possible after delivery	☐
71. Assists the new parents in getting to know their infant	☐	Does not assist the new parents in getting to know their infant or assists inappropriately	☐

learn the appropriate behavior. The instructors were told that I was to do the scoring after all of the checklists had been submitted, but they were not informed of the method to be used in arriving at a score.

RESULTS
Owing to the small number of students who can typically be accommodated in a labor and delivery unit at any one time for clinical experience, only a total of 79 usable behavior checklists was obtained from the four sample schools. An additional number of checklists were not usable because they were incomplete, were done retrospectively, or were apparently evaluating a student's performance over a period of days rather than for a period of time on a particular day.

SCORING THE CHECKLIST
The decision was made to award two points for each acceptable behavior, one point for each behavior not observed or with a zero (0) marked, and no points for those behaviors checked as unacceptable. The rationale for giving one point to the zero responses was that some instructors may have used that "category" rather than check the behavior as unacceptable, which might have been interpreted by the scorer as reflecting either poor teaching or poor evaluating technique.

In scoring the checklists, it was obvious that instructors had checked a disproportionate number of behaviors as zero. Quite frequently there was a written comment explaining the zero to signify either "not observed," or, commonly, "Not required of students in this school." In retrospect, it would have been desirable to have an additional category, "not appropriate." This category could then have meant that it was either not the practice in that hospital or that students were not taught to do it or were not expected to do it. Such a category would probably have lowered the number of zero responses while increasing knowledge of the behaviors not expected of students in the situation studied. Those activities or behaviors marked with a zero would thus have been limited to those not demonstrated by the student when he or she was being observed. There are also instances when an evaluator is unable to observe the student's performance due to myriad circumstances—truly "not observed"— and in some other instances is not able to judge whether or not the student's performance is acceptable, though this latter circumstance is not likely to occur when behaviors are explicitly stated.

It was also clear that a large number of students were not following patients from the time of admission through the first hour after delivery. This conclusion was drawn from the fact that the first three pages of the four-page checklist contained many behaviors that were marked as observed while the last page, representing patient care following delivery, were mostly marked as not being observed. This finding was not particularly surprising since some women's labors are rather long. If a student has one such follow-through experience in the course of her education, it is about the most one can expect. The tabulation of all of the instructors' observations for each behavior is given in Table 4-1.

SCORES OBTAINED

The highest possible score on the Criterion Behaviors Checklist was 142, since there were 71 behaviors included in the checklist. The range of scores for the total sample was 68 to 133, the mean score was approximately 111, and the standard deviation was 13.23. The range of scores within each of the four schools in the sample varied considerably, from a difference of 31 to a difference of 60. Three of the four schools had means that varied little as contrasted with the one where the mean was approximately 12 points more than the highest of the other three. The standard deviations varied considerably from a low of 9.12 to a high of 17.08. The frequency distributions for the checklist scores are given in Table 4-2, and the range of scores, mean scores, standard deviations, and sample sizes are presented in Table 4-3.

RELIABILITY OF THE CHECKLIST

As with any new measurement tool, an estimate of the reliability of the instrument should be made. The basic formula for calculating the reliability based on internal consistency is coefficient alpha [27]. The reliability coefficient for the Behaviors Checklist, the coefficient alpha, was .899, which was surprisingly high.

CORRELATIONS BETWEEN FILM TEST SCORES AND SCORES ON THE CHECKLIST

Pearson product-moment correlations were calculated for the Behaviors Checklist scores with each of the subscores and for the total film test scores (discussed in Chap. 3) by schools as well as for the total sample. None of the correlations were significant at the .05 level (it should be remembered that sample size was small).

It had been theorized that Subscore A scores (items based on actual film content) would correlate more significantly with the checklist scores than would either Subscore B scores or total test scores. The coefficients of correlations between the Behaviors Checklist scores and each of the subscore scores and the total scores are given in Table 4-4. The relationship of scores on the Behaviors Checklist to those on the test is shown in Table 4-5, a scatter diagram.

The data were also analyzed through the use of a stepwise multiple regression technique. Multiple correlations of the dependent variable, the Behaviors Checklist, with the independent variables, the five test parts, were computed but none of the multiple R's were significant.

A result that was most disappointing though not surprising was the failure to obtain significant correlations between the scores for Subscore A test items and the Behaviors Checklist scores. It had been theorized that students scoring high on the Subscore A items would also score high in performance. Since only 79 checklists were submitted out of the 267

Table 4-1. Tabulation of Observations by Instructors Using the Criterion Behaviors Checklist (N = 79)

No. of Behavior	Acceptable	Unacceptable	Not Observed[a]
1	72	3	4
2	70	3	6
3	16	0	63
4	36	2	39[b]
5	65	9	5
6	72	3	3[b]
7	67	1	11
8	46	7	26
9	47	9	23
10	27	12	40
11	24	12	43
12	75	0	4
13	60	0	19
14	75	3	1
15	40	1	38
16	18	0	61
17	24	0	55
18	72	4	3
19	72	5	2
20	68	4	7
21	66	9	4
22	52	2	25
23	19	1	59
24	54	2	17[b]
25	72	2	5
26	53	0	25[b]
27	42	1	36
28	50	0	29
29	25	0	54
30	30	3	46
31	62	2	15
32	62	1	16
33	39	0	40
34	52	1	26
35	4	0	68[b]
36	54	6	18[b]
37	54	0	25
38	78	1	0
39	30	0	41[b]
40	38	0	41
41	59	3	17
42	60	2	17
43	6	0	66[b]
44	10	0	61[b]
45	8	0	63[b]
46	43	0	27[b]
47	24	0	48[b]
48	16	0	56[b]
49	60	0	19

Table 4-1 (continued)

No. of Behavior	Acceptable	Unacceptable	Not Observed[a]
50	64	0	15
51	64	0	15
52	64	0	15
53	54	0	25
54	14	0	57[b]
55	14	0	57[b]
56	56	2	21
57	52	0	27
58	50	0	29
59	71	0	8
60	68	0	10[b]
61	21	0	58
62	69	0	10
63	67	0	12
64	72	0	7
65	58	0	21
66	54	0	24[b]
67	30	0	49
68	67	0	12
69	66	0	13
70	25	0	54
71	25	0	54

[a]This column covers those behaviors at which a zero was placed.
[b]Totals may not add up to 79 because for these behaviors a comment such as "Not required" was used rather than a checkmark.

Table 4-2. Frequency Distributions of Behaviors Checklist Scores from Four Sample Schools

Checklist Score	School				No. of Checklists in Sample
	1	2	3	4	
132–135	4				4
128–131	5	1			6
124–127		3			3
120–123	4	1	1	2	8
116–119	7		2	1	10
112–115	10		1		11
108–111	3		3	1	7
104–107	3	2	2	1	8
100–103	1	2	1	2	6
96–99	1	1	2	3	7
92–95		3			3
88–91			2	1	3
84–87			1		1
80–83		1			1
Below 80		1			1
Total	38	15	15	11	79

Table 4-3. Range of Scores, Mean Scores, and Standard Deviations for
Four Sample Schools on Behaviors Checklist

Variable	School				Total for Sample
	1	2	3	4	
Range of scores	99–133	68–128	84–123	89–120	68–133
Mean score	117.71	104.80	104.33	105.27	110.99
Standard deviation	9.12	17.08	11.08	10.14	13.23
Sample size	38	15	15	11	79

Table 4-4. Correlation Coefficients Between Test Subscores, Total Test
Scores, and Behaviors Checklist Scores, by School

School	No. of Checklists Used	Subscore A[a]	Subscore B[b]	Total Test Scores
1	38	.128	-.098	.008
2	15	.466	.272	.470
3	15	-.138	.322	.115
4	11	.303	-.243	.045
Total	79	.210	.037	.153

[a]Those items for which seeing the film was necessary in order to answer.
[b]Those items that can probably be answered without seeing the film.
Note: None of the correlations were significant.

students who took the film test, however, the other 188 students' scores,
had they been available, might well have greatly affected the correlations.

In addition to the small sample size involved in these correlations, mention must be made of the fact that *many* instructors in the four different
schools did the required evaluations of performance. Even though the
instructions were the same and the same form was used by all, the other
variables involved in evaluation were not controllable. Although checklists
were supposedly submitted for students currently receiving their clinical
experience, it is conceivable that instructor bias was operative in the selection of students for evaluation for the purposes of the study. The fact that
the correlations (cognitive test scores with performance scores) were not
significant was in keeping with many other studies—both in nursing and
in medicine—reporting comparable results. Representative of such studies
are those by Dunn [6], Price and associates [31], and Levine and McGuire
[21].

Another possible explanation for the failure to obtain significant correlations between the checklist scores and the film test scores lies in the difference in content covered in each tool. While all of the content pertained
to obstetric nursing, the checklist was broader in scope than the test,
covering all of the measures that patients require during labor and delivery
as well as those that may be obligatory in some institutions. In addition,

Table 4-5. *Scatter Diagram for Behaviors Checklist Scores and Total Test Scores for Sample (N = 79)*

	Behaviors Checklist Score																
Test Score	68/71	72/75	76/79	80/83	84/87	88/91	92/95	96/99	100/103	104/107	108/111	112/115	116/119	120/123	124/127	128/131	132/133
44–45																	
42–43																	
40–41								2								1	
38–39															1		
36–37						2		1	2	1	2	2	5	1	1	1	
34–35								1		2	2	4		2			
32–33						1	1	2	2	2		2	2	2	1	2	1
30–31									2	1	1	1	1		1	1	3
28–29							1							1			
26–27	1			1									1		1		
24–25										1		1					
22–23					1												
20–21							1										

the checklist included the measures generally utilized in patient care during the early postpartum period. The test based on the film was limited in content and pertained only to those aspects of labor and delivery actually presented. Although the content of the film test was deliberately extended to make it more representative of the constellation of knowledge and behaviors relevant to obstetric nursing, it was impossible to force content such as postpartum care into the test and still preserve its face validity.

DISCUSSION OF THE FINDINGS

Although no one criticized the checklist per se, I feel it might have listed only the acceptable behaviors, with two columns provided for checking whether or not the behavior was acceptable. Since the physical appearance of an evaluation tool is likely to influence the degree to which it is used, the original Criterion Behaviors Checklist was printed on both sides of the paper, resulting in a two-page rather than a four-page tool. The design of a two-page tool rather than a four-page tool was an attempt to make the tool appear less detailed and cumbersome.

The results obtained from the checklists were a little surprising and very disappointing. Since the behaviors were deemed explicit in defining what was acceptable behavior and what was not, the addition of comments by some instructors alongside some of the behaviors was unexpected. Some words were crossed out, others were added, but what was particularly disappointing were the comments "Tries" or "Sometimes" next to an acceptable behavior. The observation of clinical performance was supposed to be done during one clinical laboratory experience, but it was obvious from this that some of the instructors had used the checklist as a cumulative evaluation form, while others had used it retrospectively. Therefore it can be concluded that faculty using the tool were unfamiliar with both the format and the method.

The faculty member in charge of the obstetric experience in one program did tell me that since the evaluation method in use in their school differed so greatly from what was being asked of them by the Behaviors Checklist, she would make the special effort necessary to have some of the students evaluated according to the checklist. A sample of that institution's clinical evaluation form was made available. It consisted of only five words with space provided for instructors' comments. Among the words listed were "attitude," "planning," and "intervention." No guidelines indicating how the tool was to be used accompanied the form, and it appeared to be a terminal or summative one, since space was provided for dates and a clinical practice grade. Most surprising was the fact that a grade for clinical performance was awarded the student on the basis of that tool. This very subjective and ambiguous method of evaluating clinical performance was standard in one of the Ivy League colleges of nursing in 1973.

A well-known phenomenon that frequently occurs when clinical performance is evaluated—the "halo effect"—was apparently operative with this study, too. The checklists showed evidence of this effect, in particular from the school that submitted the greatest number of them (School 1).

The lowest score on the checklist from that school was 99 as compared to the next lowest score from any other school, which was 89; and the mean score was approximately 12.5 points higher than the next highest mean. These data are given in Table 4-3. It is conceivable that some instructors marked a zero rather than marking the behavior Unacceptable. This possibility could be broadened to include their checking the Acceptable column rather than the Unacceptable one rather than saying the behavior was not observed.

Schools 3 and 4 are recognized for their excellence in preparing competent nursing practitioners at the baccalaureate level. It was not surprising to find these two schools having the highest individual test scores as well as test means. What was surprising was the fact that they also had the individuals with the lowest top scores on the Behaviors Checklist. (The mean scores and ranges of scores on the test are given in Table 3-11, the mean scores and ranges of scores on the checklist are given in Table 4-3, and the frequency distribution of the checklist scores is given in Table 4-2.) In partial explanation of this surprising fact, the method of evaluation usually used in one of the two schools was very subjective, and there was a reluctance on the part of faculty to use the Behaviors Checklist. It also appeared that the faculty, in addition to being unfamiliar with such a tool, were confusing the teaching process with the evaluating process. That is, when one is teaching the focus is on integration of content, whereas for purposes of evaluation the content *needs* to be broken down into the constituent elements. The obvious implication of these findings is that instructors need more help in the process of evaluation than they have had in graduate school.

The tabulation of instructors' ratings (see Table 4-1) was studied in relation to the two possible categories not specifically mentioned in the Checklist, Not Observed and Not Applicable. If, for example, one looks at behavior 16—"Performs the admission procedures correctly, e.g., perineal shave, enema, urine specimen," and notes that a zero was placed there for 61 students, it is fairly clear that students were not performing these procedures. Their not doing so may have been due to institutional policy, to the fact that they were not there when women were admitted to the labor and delivery suite, or to the fact that the procedures were not considered necessary to the objectives for the clinical laboratory experience. For other behaviors, such as number 23, "Encourages husband to participate in his wife's care," where a zero was listed for 59 students, it can be assumed that husbands were not present, with one possible reason being that hospital policy did not permit them to be.

On the positive side, one can, by scanning the large numbers in the Acceptable column, deduce which behaviors are expected of students and which ones they are performing. For example, behavior 14 is "Times uterine contractions accurately and at appropriate intervals"; there was only 1 student checked with a zero (not observed) at this place, 3 students performed the procedure unacceptably and 75 performed it acceptably. (I am prompted to say "Thank goodness.")

One would also question whether the students had had the opportunity to learn what they were being evaluated on. Numerous articles reveal that experiences with laboring women are hard to come by. That situation was confirmed in casual discussion with many instructors, some of whom were involved in the study and some of whom were not. Students, in fact, are considered lucky if they have one experience of caring for a woman in labor. This results, most unfortunately, in the student's learning and being evaluated concurrently.

The possibility of obtaining clinical performance evaluations for students on a particular school's form and filled out in the manner usual for its program had been considered early in the study but was rejected. Comparing any two such forms would have been impossible. Instead, the Criterion Behaviors Checklist was designed to enable such comparison. All of the instructors would at least be using the same form. In retrospect, perhaps the global clinical performance evaluations from instructors would have shed some light on what was expected of their students and, of course, on how they were evaluated. In addition, it might have been possible to compare the scores obtained on the film test with the grade assigned by the instructor on their form for clinical performance.

A point not previously mentioned is the desirability of giving the performance evaluation tool to nursing students before they are evaluated. They have the right to know the criteria used when they are evaluated. Perhaps if they are evaluated objectively, specifically, and constructively, the next generation of nurse instructors, the present students, will be better equipped for the difficult, challenging, and important task of evaluation.

THE REVISED CHECKLIST

The Criterion Behaviors Checklist that was submitted to the instructors in the study schools contained essentially the same behaviors as those contained in the revised version. Minor changes have been made to coincide with current practice in obstetric nursing. For example, the behavior "Gives breast care before mother breast-feeds her infant" has been reworded to say "Teaches breast care to the breast-feeding mother." The instructions for use of the checklist have also been revised in keeping with the new format and may be less ambiguous than those given on the original checklist. Two columns have been added: Not Observed and Not Applicable; the latter covers those behaviors that are neither applicable nor appropriate at the time the student is being observed. A major change has been the elimination of the negatively worded behaviors. Besides the fact that it might appear that such behaviors were condoned, stating the same behavior both positively and negatively makes the evaluation form appear crowded, and the appearance of an evaluation tool *is* important. A two- or three-page tool is far more likely to be used and used correctly than is a tool that is 10 or 12 pages long.

The revised checklist is shown on the following pages.

Labor and Delivery Clinical Laboratory Experience:
Criterion Behaviors Checklist

Student _____   Date of Observation _____
                                    Time of Observation _____
                                    Observer _____

Instructions: Place a ✓ mark next to the behavior observed—either it was an acceptable one or an unacceptable one. When the period of observation is ended, place a 0 in the Not Observed column for any behavior not actually demonstrated. If a behavior is either not applicable or not appropriate to the experience, mark a ✓ mark in the Not Applicable column.

Criterion Behaviors	Acceptable	Unacceptable	Not Observed	Not Applicable
Introduces self to patient				
Explains to patient how nurse will participate in her care				
Checks patient's valuables, dealing with them according to hospital policy				
Wears only a smooth-strapped watch with a second hand				
Uses language appropriate for both patient's intellectual level and emotional state when giving instructions or explanations				
Relates pertinent observations and findings promptly to the instructor				
Records observations and findings both accurately and promptly				
Elicits relevant history, including symptoms of true labor				
Finds out what patient knows about the process of labor and delivery				
Palpates patient's abdomen for fetal position before auscultation of the fetal heartbeat				

Criterion Behaviors	Acceptable	Unacceptable	Not Observed	Not Applicable	
Places fingers on patient's radial artery while listening to the fetal heartbeat					
Takes fetal heart rate after contractions, after rupture of the membranes, and after the administration of medications					
Takes patient's vital signs following the administration of medications and/or anesthesia and at appropriate intervals					
Times uterine contractions accurately and at appropriate intervals					
Explains purpose and procedure of the perineal preparation and enema before proceeding with the procedure					
Performs the admission procedures correctly, e.g., perineal shave, enema, urine specimen					
Permits patient to ambulate until her membranes rupture, according to hospital policy					
Encourages patient to breathe abdominally, deeply, and slowly during contractions in the early first stage of labor					
Encourages patient to relax between contractions					
Permits patient to express herself freely without interjection of inappropriate comments					
Alleviates patient's fears and reduces her tension to the degree possible by using appropriate means					
Keeps patient and her husband apprised of the progress of labor					
Encourages husband to participate in his wife's care					

Criterion Behaviors	Acceptable	Unacceptable	Not Observed	Not Applicable
Encourages patient to pant during contractions at the end of the first stage of labor				
Institutes measures to promote patient comfort, such as back rubs, mouth rinses, sponge baths, perineal care				
Administers oral fluids according to hospital policy				
Interprets the purpose of intravenous fluids when they are instituted, and carries out the same routine with the maternity patient as with other adult patients, e.g., monitoring rate of flow				
Assists patient with positioning to facilitate respiratory exchange, pushing efforts, and the administration of anesthetics, and to prevent postural hypotension				
Prepares and administers medications accurately				
Interprets to the patient the procedure to be used to anesthetize her				
Puts side rails up after patient has been medicated or has received an anesthetic agent				
Observes perineum for bulging and crowning				
Completely covers nose and mouth with mask when the perineum is exposed in the labor room and during delivery				
Removes mask when it is not needed and changes it when it becomes moist				

Criterion Behaviors	Acceptable	Unacceptable	Not Observed	Not Applicable
Checks the delivery room to be sure that it has all necessary equipment in readiness—sterile instruments, basins, linen, and a heated crib with resuscitation equipment				
Encourages patient to void at periodic intervals and before being taken to the delivery room				
Transfers patient from bed to stretcher and vice versa safely				
Completely covers hair with scrub cap in the delivery room				
Places patient in lithotomy position on the delivery table, putting both legs in stirrups at the same time				
Restrains patient's hands if indicated				
Checks fetal heart rate at least every 5 minutes				
Encourages patient to push with each contraction during the second stage				
Cleanses perineum according to hospital policy, using aseptic technique				
Accurately administers medications, e.g., oxytocics, during delivery or after delivery of the placenta depending on physician's orders				
Disposes of placenta according to hospital policy				
Records observations and other required information accurately and promptly, e.g., time of delivery of infant and of placenta				
Evaluates the infant using the Apgar scoring system at one minute and five minutes after birth				

Criterion Behaviors	Acceptable	Unacceptable	Not Observed	Not Applicable	
Notifies instructor of an Apgar score below 7					
Performs those procedures dictated by hospital policy for newborns, e.g., weighing, temperature by rectum, instillation of eye medication, identification of baby and mother, administration of vitamin K					
Keeps infant warm					
Appraises infant quickly for gross anomalies					
Keeps infant positioned to promote patency of the airway with drainage of mucus					
Shows infant to his mother after wiping his face and head of blood and secretions					
Teaches breast care to the breast-feeding mother					
Assists the breast-feeding mother in helping her infant to nurse					
Checks infant's identification with the mother before the baby is transferred to the nursery					
Transfers infant to the nursery according to hospital policy					
Removes patient's legs from the stirrups at the same time					
Applies perineal pad; examines it and the pad under the patient every 15 minutes for amount of lochia					
Notifies instructor if lochia is excessive					
Keeps a hand on the uterine fundus for the first hour after delivery					

Criterion Behaviors	Acceptable	Unacceptable	Not Observed	Not Applicable
Massages uterine fundus correctly if boggy				
Notifies instructor if uterine fundus is boggy				
Takes vital signs at specified intervals				
Encourages patient to void, noting amount				
Gives perineal care after patient uses the bedpan for the first time postpartum				
Bathes patient after delivery, partially or completely, as warranted				
Changes gown and bed linens as necessary				
Examines the episiotomy for oozing and hematomas				
Arranges for the new family to be together as soon as possible after delivery				
Assists the new parents in getting to know their infant				

REFERENCES

1. Araneta, N. C., and Miller, C. L. Philosophical systems of weighting clinical performance in nursing. *Int. J. Nurs. Stud.* 7:235, 1970.
2. Bernhardt, J., and Schuette, L. P.E.T.—A method of evaluating professional nurse performance. *J. Nurs. Admin.* 5:18, 1975.
3. Burke, R. J., and Goodale, J. G. New Way to Rate Nurse Performance. In S. Stone, et al. (Eds.), *Management for Nurses.* St. Louis: C. V. Mosby, 1976.
4. Campbell, J. P., Dunnette, M., Arvey, R., and Hellervik, L. The development and evaluation of behaviorally based rating scales. *J. Appl. Psychol.* 57:15, 1973.
5. del Bueno, D. J. The cost of competency. *J. Nurs. Admin.* 5:16, 1975.
6. Dunn, M. A. Development of an instrument to measure nursing performance. *Nurs. Res.* 19:502, 1970.
7. Dyer, E. D. Nurse Performance Description: Criteria, Predictors, and Correlates. Ed.D. dissertation, University of Utah, 1967.
8. Dyer, E. D. Nurse Performance Description: Criteria, Predictors, and Correlates. In *Fifth Nursing Research Conference* (New Orleans: March 3–5, 1969). New York: American Nurses' Association, 1971.
9. Fivars, G., and Gosnell, D. *Nursing Evaluation: The Problem and the Process: The Critical Incident Technique.* New York: Macmillan, 1966.
10. Gudmundsen, A. Teaching psychomotor skills. *J. Nurs. Educ.* 14:23, 1975.
11. Haar, L. P., and Hicks, J. R. Performance appraisal: Derivation of effective assessment tools. *J. Nurs. Admin.* 6:20, 1976.
12. Hayter, J. An approach to laboratory evaluation. *J. Nurs. Educ.* 12:17, 1973.
13. Heins, M., Hawk, T., Busch, J., DeRidder, L., Flitter, H., and Ray, J. *Evaluation and Prediction of Clinical Performance in a School of Nursing.* Knoxville, Tenn.: St. Mary's Memorial Hospital School of Nursing, 1971.
14. Hilliard, M. *Orientation and Evaluation of the Professional Nurse.* St. Louis: C. V. Mosby, 1974.
15. Hoose, D. C. A model for a nursing media center. *Nurs. Outlook* 24:104, 1976.
16. Infante, M. S. *The Clinical Laboratory in Nursing Education.* New York: John Wiley, 1975.
17. Johnson, C. A., and Hurley, R. S. Design and use of an instrument to evaluate students' clinical performance. *J. Am. Diet. Assoc.* 68:450, 1976.
18. Klimoski, R. J., and London, M. Role of the rater in performance appraisal. *J. Appl. Psychol.* 59:445, 1974.
19. Krumme, U. S. The case for criterion-referenced measurement. *Nurs. Outlook* 23:764, 1975.
20. Lenburg, C. B. The external degree in nursing: The promise fulfilled. *Nurs. Outlook* 24:422, 1976.
21. Levine, H. G., and McGuire, C. H. Rating habitual performance in graduate medical education. *J. Med. Educ.* 46:306, 1971.
22. Litwack, L. A system for evaluation. *Nurs. Outlook* 24:45, 1976.
23. Marshall, J. R., and Schau, E. An evaluation process for nursing assistants. *J. Nurs. Admin.* 6:37, 1976.
24. McGuire, C. A Proposed Model for the Evaluation of Teaching. In *The Evaluation of Teaching,* A Report of the Second Pi Lambda Theta Catena, Washington, 1967.
25. National League for Nursing Council of Associate Degree Programs.

Preparing the Associate Degree Graduate. (Papers presented at a Preparing the Associate Degree Graduate Workshop, October, 1976, Cincinnati, Ohio.) New York: National League for Nursing, 1977.

26. Nichols, E. G., and Heydman, A. H. Staff participation in student evaluation. *Supervisor Nurs.* 7:74, 1976.
27. Nunnally, J. C. *Psychometric Theory.* New York: McGraw-Hill, 1967.
28. Pearson, B. D. A model for clinical evaluation. *Nurs. Outlook* 23:232, 1975.
29. Peterson, C., Connelly, S., DePew, C., Cowden, M., and Mayer, G. *Teaching and Evaluating Synthesis in an Associate Degree Nursing Program—a Developmental Experience.* New York: National League for Nursing, 1975.
30. Petrovich, S. Evaluation Based on Philosophy and Objectives, Conceptual Framework, Curriculum Threads and Course Objectives. In *Preparing the Associate Degree Graduate.* New York: National League for Nursing, 1977.
31. Price, P. B., Taylor, C., Nelson, D., Lewis, E., Loughmiller, G., Mathiesen, R., Murray, S., and Maxwell, J. *Measurement and Predictors of Physician Performance: Two Decades of Intermittently Sustained Research.* Salt Lake City: Aaron Press, 1971.
32. *Some Objective Approaches to Evaluation: Case Presentations* (League Exchange No. 98). New York: National League for Nursing, 1972.
33. Tate, B. L. *A Method for Rating the Proficiency of the Hospital General Staff Nurse.* New York: National League for Nursing, 1964.
34. Tate, B. L. Evaluating the nurse's clinical performance. *Nurs. Outlook* 10:35, 1962.
35. Tate, B. L. *Test of a Nursing Performance Evaluation Instrument.* New York: National League for Nursing, 1964.
36. Thorndike, R. L., and Hagen, E. P. *Measurement and Evaluation in Psychology and Education* (4th ed.). New York: John Wiley, 1977.
37. Tower, J. B., and Vosburgh, P. M. Development of a rating scale to measure learning in clinical dietetics. I. Theoretical considerations and method of construction. *J. Am. Diet. Assoc.* 68:440, 1976.
38. Trammel, C. K. The Development of Performance Criteria to Assist in the Evaluation of Clinical Performance in a Beginning Medical-Surgical Nursing Course. Ed.D. dissertation, University of Alabama, 1974.
39. Vosburgh, P. M., Tower, J., Peckos, P., and Mason, M. Development of a rating scale to measure learning in clinical dietetics. II. Pilot test. *J. Am. Diet. Assoc.* 68:446, 1976.
40. Wandelt, M. A., and Slater Stewart, D. *Slater Nursing Competencies Rating Scale.* New York: Appleton-Century-Crofts, 1975.
41. Wilson, M. A. *Equivalency Evaluation in Development of Health Practitioners.* Thorofare, N.J.: Charles B. Slack, 1976.
42. Wise, B. B. A taxonomy approach. . . implications for performance. *J. Continu. Educ. Nurs.* 3:9, 1972.
43. Wood, L. A., and Rambo, B. J. (Eds.). *Nursing Skills for Allied Health Services* (2nd ed.). Philadelphia: W. B. Saunders, 1975.
44. Woolley, A. S. The long and tortured history of clinical evaluation. *Nurs. Outlook* 25:308, 1977.
45. Zedeck, S., and Baker, H. T. Nursing performance as measured by behavioral expectation scales: A multitrait—multirater analysis. *Organ. Behav. Hum. Perf.* 7:457, 1972.

5. Use of Videotape Recordings in Evaluation

Television has become a way of life for millions of people, with even toddlers asking to see particular programs such as "Sesame Street." Elementary schools offer homebound students opportunities for keeping up with their peers by means of closed-circuit television and provide for participation by the child via a two-way communication system. Courses in audiovisual media that are now offered beginning in the early school years include the making of movies and videotapes and their design and use. We are all familiar with closed-circuit surveillance systems in hospitals, banks, elevators, apartment houses, and stores. Staff education programs in hospitals have provided lectures by prominent people or allowed us to "look over the shoulder" of an eminent surgeon performing a procedure destined to make medical history. If there was some reason why it wasn't possible to attend that viewing, arrangements could be made to see it at another, more convenient time.

HOW HAVE VIDEOTAPES BEEN USED?

The use of television for teaching purposes has been and continues to be widely used. It has been utilized for training and updating skills and providing knowledge in industry as well as in hospitals. Colleges have employed it in a wide variety of ways, including the teaching of Shakespeare [28] and cultural phenomena in a sociology course [24].

Another instructional use of television has been to teach dietitians, their ancillary workers, and other allied health professionals those subjects related to nutrition and food service. This cooperative effort involved 10 agencies within a community and included the use of specially prepared videotapes as well as some that were commercially prepared [29].

It has also been used moderately in the nursing field. In a continuing education program for staff nurses clinical simulations have been videotaped and used to teach the nursing process [26]. Videotapes have been used in a nurse-practitioner course to assist nurses with self-cognition of their history-taking skills [27]. In an associate degree nursing program, videotapes of the students' clinical performance have been used to help them to "sharpen their observational and psychomotor skills and to share varied experiences" [25].

The use of videotape recordings for the purpose of evaluation has almost kept pace with its teaching uses. In the early sixties, Griffin and his colleagues [8] reported on the use of closed-circuit television by instructors to monitor the performance of nursing students. One instructor could observe several students giving care in different areas of the hospital.

Several programs for registered nurse students have used videotapes of nursing performance in various ways. In a graduate course on teaching strategies, a student's teaching performance is videotaped and immediately replayed. The student, the student's classmates, and the instructor all rate the performance using a prepared rating scale [3]. In contrast to most challenge examinations, which usually are paper-and-pencil tests, a novel approach was used in designing an examination for registered nurse students who wished to challenge a course in interpersonal relations and the therapeutic use of self. The students were videotaped while counseling a "client"—a friend, classmate, or patient; they then evaluated themselves while being rated by at least two instructors [6]. (The rating guide used in this project to assess performance contains 20 behaviors or statements that were to be assigned a score of zero to three. It also contains behaviors difficult if not impossible to assess, e.g., "Degree of genuiness of self." It illustrates some of the problems with rating scales that were raised in Chap. 4.)

Interpersonal skills were also the focus for evaluation in another program for registered nurse students. Brief videotapes of patient situations were shown to which the students had to write their responses. What is particularly interesting about this test is that three levels of responses were established in three categories. The levels of responses were (1) most therapeutic, (2) appropriate, and (3) least appropriate. The categories were (1) What would you say?, (2) What would you do?, and (3) Give principles or the rationale for the response given and the action taken [23].

The use of videotapes for evaluating the performance of medical students has also been reported. Hess [10] was concerned about the lack of inter-rater reliability in judging the ability of medical students to relate to patients in a medical setting; he used videotapes with two different rating systems in an attempt to discover the more reliable method of the two for rating students' performance. One of the systems used effective-ineffective behaviors along a 10-point continuum, while the other used a system of interaction-analysis behaviors reported in units. In addition to the three physician-raters, self-evaluations and peer evaluations were included in the study. Hess found the more reliable method to be the one that used the interaction-analysis procedure. One of the advantages of the self-confrontation methodology, Hess reported, is that it helps students to change their behavior in the affective domain.

The clinical competence of medical students in the field of pediatrics was the focus of a study by Turner and associates [30]. They built upon the work of Hess, particularly in relation to the scoring method. Although the findings generally agreed with those of Hess, they concluded with the statement that "perhaps the videotape method should be explored further as a tool in studying clinical performance [30]."

Other uses of videotape include the training of observers in the use of a checklist or rating scale with the intent being to establish greater inter-rater reliability and therefore more reliable ratings [2, 10, 30]. Self-confrontation, with videotape recording, of one's teaching performance and the effects of a trained critic on self-devaluation were the bases of another study that used military instructor–trainees [31]. The dependent variable was the presence or absence of a critique by the instructor prior to the videotape being replayed and the self-rating. A 7-point rating scale listing 7 teaching behaviors was used.

Videotape Techniques in Psychiatric Training and Treatment [1], an excellent book edited by M. M. Berger, reveals a great deal about the wide applicability of videotapes in yet another area. Interestingly, this book contains reports of the use of videotapes in psychiatry in the mid-sixties; one wonders if there have been any advances in their use since. In addition to the recording of actual patient behaviors, simulation techniques with role-playing were used to serve both teaching and evaluation purposes.

What has been presented here is an overview of the uses of videotape recordings in education. In all probability, I've only just skimmed the surface of the field. What one does surmise from a review of the literature is that video is in its infancy and that "It has not been quite invented yet [20]." Advances in the development of equipment continue to be made, however, that will in time further facilitate the recording and replaying of videotapes. Color cassettes are in the process of refinement and video discs that can be played like a phonograph record are even now in the works.

ADVANTAGES AND DISADVANTAGES OF VIDEOTAPE RECORDINGS

There are presently many advantages to the use of videotape recordings in the field of education as compared to other media. Among the advantages are the following:

1. The instant playback capability is probably its chief advantage; it is certainly more quickly available than are movies.
2. The equipment is easy to operate and the videotapes are easy to work with.
3. Special lighting is not usually needed since video cameras are effective at low light intensities.
4. It is much less expensive than film, and this includes the video equipment.
5. Videotapes can be replayed as often as necessary.
6. Running time of the videotape can be compressed to fit a specific period, e.g., a class period.
7. The closed-circuit feature makes it especially useful for restricted viewings, e.g., in a hospital.
8. It eliminates the need for repetitive teaching.
9. Videotapes are erasable and therefore reusable.
10. More continuous filming time is possible with video equipment.
11. Video does not present problems with synchronization of sound because it is automatic.

Among the disadvantages that are relevant to their use in education are the following:

1. When viewing the performance of a person on videotape, there is no saving of time. In fact, more than one viewing may be necessary.
2. Students who have not been exposed to the use of videotapes in education may have difficulty in accepting them as teaching devices rather than as an entertainment medium.
3. The instructors, the student's peers, and the other players in the videotape recordings may be subject to varying degrees of criticism by the students who view the tapes.
4. If the videotape is being used for teaching purposes, the pace may be too rapid for students. Koch [12] states that about 90 minutes of classroom instruction is covered in about 45 minutes of a teleclass.
5. Many instructors are not familiar with the operation of video equipment, but the same thing might be said of movie equipment. (This is a relatively easy problem to solve since more and more workshops are being offered around the country in the use of such equipment and in the making of videotapes for use in education.)

USING VIDEOTAPE RECORDINGS IN EVALUATION

As has been documented earlier, videotapes of performance have been used for the purpose of evaluation. The evaluations have been done by any one or more of the following persons: the student whose performance has been recorded, the student's peers, and one or more instructors. Videotapes of a performer unknown to the group can also be critiqued by a total group. Rating scales or checklists have been used in some of the projects and should be used when assessing the videotaped performance since such scales or checklists will direct the observations to be made (see Chap. 4 for a sample of a checklist that could be adapted for just such a purpose). If one is not sure whether or not a particular behavior was demonstrated, the videotape can be rewound to the point in question and reviewed, and as often as necessary. (One caution must be voiced again: there will be no saving of evaluator time in the viewing of videotaped performances!)

In addition to the use of videotapes in the evaluation of clinical performance, they can be used as the stimulus for a test in the cognitive domain, much as the film *Birth Day—Through the Eyes of the Mother* was used as the stimulus for the sample test in Chapter 3. An advantage of the videotapes is that they can be short (only several minutes long), depicting small segments of a patient-nurse interaction and focused on a specific fact, principle, or concept. Students can be asked to evaluate the plan for a patient's care or evaluate the implementation of that plan or both. The level of the student can also be taken into consideration, adding complexity to the patient-care situation when it is indicated. The students can be asked to supply better responses to patients' queries than did the nurses in the videotape. Questions can also be designed to assess objectives in the affective domain. Much of the design of the videotape and the questions that are dependent on it are a function of the creativity of the instructor-developer. The sample test at the end of this chapter, which uses videotaped vignettes as the stimuli for the test questions, is a demonstration of that kind of creativity by faculty in a baccalaureate nursing program.

Another advantage of videotapes for testing purposes is the fact that they can be viewed under ordinary lighting conditions and in fact may need some artificial light, which could facilitate the test-taking process. Lights will not have to be turned on and off depending on whether the students are viewing the videotape or responding to the questions. One point that is particularly important is that there should be enough monitors so that students can have an unobstructed view of the videotapes. There is no formula as to the number of students per monitor since it depends in part on the size of the monitor.

MAKING A VIDEOTAPE FOR USE IN EVALUATION

What follows are some of the many considerations involved as well as some of the decisions that will need to be made before undertaking such a project. It is not meant to be, nor can it be, the definitive work on the subject (I leave that to the experts). However, I hope that by discussing some of the components of videotaping, certain possible pitfalls will not come as a surprise and will therefore be more easily managed.

If the decision has been made to make a videotape, consideration should have been given to the costs of producing the product. The fact that videotapes are less expensive to produce than films will probably not be specific enough for budgetary requirements. Because of improvements and new developments in the field, it is senseless to quote current prices; for example, a color camera that at last report costs $5,000 for a self-contained portable unit may be less than half that price within a year. Videotape that now costs $25 for one hour of shooting time may be just a few dollars next year. What will have to be done is to check prices of all of the necessary equipment at the outset of the project. Since many colleges and universities have audiovisual departments, a ready source of information is personnel in these departments. Commercial enterprises are also more than willing to assist in a school's venture into videotape recordings. Books and periodicals in the field are also useful in locating avenues of assistance; for example, 32 resource organizations are listed in *The Videotape Book* by Michael Murray [20].

As with any test or audiovisual medium, one needs to decide on the purpose(s) and the expected outcomes (terminal objectives, if you will) of the material. It should be obvious that the audience needs to be not only kept in mind during the design period but specified. Although questions at the lower levels of the cognitive domain can certainly be designed, the use of audiovisual media makes the testing of the higher levels of the cognitive domain easier; for example, essay questions are particularly useful for tapping knowledge at the synthesis level.

Subject matter to be included and tested should probably be discussed concurrently with the purposes and anticipated outcomes. What sample from the universe of content should be included? Is it a representative

sample? Is the extent of the sample realistic in terms of the time constraints? A word of caution: start small, tackle a circumscribed portion of
a course. Don't start with something like "The Care of Patients with Acute
Cardiovascular Disorders."

A next step should be a decision about who is to do the actual filming or
taping. Are audiovisual experts available in the college? Will they assist
nurse faculty in the process? Are they available for consultation? If there
is no such person on the staff, perhaps an outside audiovisual consultant
could be contacted to assist in the various phases of the project.

A script is essential in order to ensure that only relevant action and
dialogue are included. Although unnecessary material can be edited out,
it is much simpler and more economical to start with the desired content.
A scenario may be more workable than a script if it is not necessary that
every word be precise or that every movement be specified. It is sometimes
desirable to have the actors improvise an encounter, such as one between a
patient and a nurse. The resulting scene would then lend itself to criticism
about what was said and done and what might have been better to say and
do. Much written material is usually organized so that there is first an
introduction, followed by the body of content, and then a summary, and
so it is with a script. Such an organization is essential for a teaching videotape or film but may not be necessary or even desirable for a "testing"
videotape or film. What may be wanted in that case is an incident to which
examinees are to respond. Organization of the script depends on the purpose, the objectives, and the test questions that are to be written.

The person responsible for writing the script should probably be the one
most knowledgeable about the subject matter. It could, of course, be
written by someone knowledgeable about script-writing, but content
would then need to be scrutinized by an expert or a panel of experts. If a
nursing faculty member writes the script, it should also be reviewed by
others on the faculty. Such a review can rectify some of the early "bugs."

There are any number of books that can help in the script-writing process, those on film-making as well as those that pertain to videotapes. A
number of possibly useful books on film-making are listed in a separate
bibliography at the end of Chapter 3. Some books on videotape recording
are listed within the references at the end of this chapter. When the time
comes to actually write a script, there may be more and newer books on
the market, so it would be well to check the library or a book store. Audiovisual experts within the college may also be very helpful in directing you
to an appropriate reference.

Along with other preparations for making the videotape, consideration
should be given to who will play the parts. Will professional actors be
hired? The availability of funds may determine whether or not professional
actors can be engaged, however. Will faculty assume the roles of patients,
staff, and the other required parts? Will some of the students do the acting?
One of the negative aspects of having faculty portray various roles is that
the students or staff may not identify them as the characters they are
playing but rather as the faculty they really are. Additionally, perfor-

mances may not win an Academy Award and therefore too much attention would be devoted to criticizing the performance rather than to attending to the content. A good solution might be to use drama students, if available, since they are likely to derive some benefits by doing so: practice, as well as satisfaction from assisting in such a project. They also can benefit from the videotapes in terms of evaluating their own performance [6]. Whatever the ultimate decision, the actors should be lined up, and a commitment should be made by them to follow through with the venture. At about the same time, a tentative schedule for rehearsals can be set up. Thompson and her associates [29] give this general rule of thumb: for every minute of the final product, two hours in preproduction time are required. A 15-minute videotape would therefore require approximately 30 hours of preparation.

A decision should be made as to where the actual taping will be done. If at all possible, rehearsals—and especially the dress rehearsal—should take place at that place. Much depends on the subject matter and purpose of the tape. Some videotapes will lend themselves to being taped in a classroom, while others may need a studio. If it is needed, a simulated laboratory can be set up and the taping can be done there. A hospital unit may be necessary, again depending on what is to be accomplished.

If a real patient is to be used, permission will need to be obtained from him or her in order to protect all involved (permission is needed from the parents of a minor and sometimes from the hospital or school administration). The hospital or school administrator should probably be contacted regarding legal requirements within the institution. Also, if professional actors are used, contracts may be necessary.

Soon after the script has been written, reviewed, and edited, the test questions and answers should be written by the faculty members responsible for the subject matter. Peer review of the questions and answers is also strongly recommended. The questions and answers will have to be reviewed once the videotapes are finished, but it is essential to write them at this point so they will be ready for that review.

When sufficient practice has taken place so that it appears everyone has memorized his lines, if this is indicated (some videotaped sessions need to be improvised because of their purpose), and "it looks good," the time has come to shoot. For some novice performers, there will be that initial stage fright or camera fright, and for some it will persist. Self-consciousness is not an uncommon reaction. For others, all will probably go well, almost as if they've been doing it all their lives.

A director should be assigned the job of overseeing production, of pulling the whole act together. What a director is likely to see in toto is apt to be far different from what each of the players envisions. The first taping may be thought of as a "dry run" and immediately following it, the recording can be replayed so that each performer can see what was good or not so good about his performance and what will need to be altered, and, of course, the director will do the same. After this viewing and any necessary directions for replaying the parts have been given, the videotape can be reshot. This last phase may need to be repeated until all are satisfied with the product. The marvelous part about using videotapes is that the tapes are erasable and can be used over and over again.

Some of the problems run into, for example, redundant action or speech, can be remedied by editing the tape already shot, making repeated shooting unnecessary; much depends on the expert assistance available. The editing process also can include the insertion of such things as a sound track, visuals such as titles or slides, and other special effects if these are desirable and indicated.

When the tape is satisfactory, the faculty will now need to view it in relation to the questions previously written. The following questions are among the ones that the faculty should be directing themselves to during this review.

1. Does the videotape provide all the stimuli necessary to answer the questions?
2. Is there footage included that should be edited out, i.e., material that might be misleading or might confuse the students, as well as taking additional time to show?
3. Do the questions "speak" to the videotape? (As was pointed out in Chap. 3, some test questions do not require the stimulus of the film or videotape, and if they do not, it is an uneconomical use of time, energy, and money to include them.)

On the basis of this viewing, modifications may need to be made in the questions and possibly in the answers. Faculty should make any necessary changes and then view the videotape again on the basis of the revised questions and answers. Such a review may need to be repeated until all the final products are satisfactory.

When the examination has gained the approval of the faculty, it should be tried out experimentally with a small group of subjects. Although it is desirable to administer the test to a group of students comparable to those for whom the test was designed, it might be tried out with faculty members who were not involved in its design. Some valuable information may be gained from such an administration, not the least of which is clarity.

Ideally, the test should then be administered to the comparable group of students. The students should be told the purpose of the administration and that the results will not be reflected or count in any way in their course grades. Again, the try-out will provide answers to questions such as the following, thus providing information that will be useful in making any revisions.

1. Did students have enough time to answer the questions?
2. Were the instructions clear?
3. Was the videotape shown often enough?
4. What were their reactions to taking this type of test?

In looking at the answers the sample of students provided, consider the following:

1. Were they in keeping with what was expected?
2. Did they include additional correct information?
3. Did a large number of students get a particular question wrong? If so, take a look at the question. Is it clear? Is there anything ambiguous about it? Was it taught or discussed in class, or were students expected to gain this information outside of class?
4. Did the scoring procedure previously established work?
5. Did the "better" students do best on the test?

Following the analyses of the directions for administration, the questions and answers, and the scoring procedure, make any necessary revisions before using the videotape test with the group of students for whom it was intended.

As soon as this videotape is in use, faculty should be thinking about new simulations that would lend themselves to this method of testing. As with any test, some students are likely to share information about a test's content with their peers so that after a test has been in use for a time, it is no longer testing very much except memory. New situations should therefore be developed to replace the older ones. The old simulations can then be used for teaching purposes, or as a sample test to acquaint students with the method so they will know what's expected of them.

Although the process of developing a videotape test is time-consuming, so is every reliable and valid test. Perhaps this approach to evaluation will offer not only diversity but will be especially useful in assessing knowledge not possible by written multiple-choice questions, in particular, knowledge at the synthesis level of the cognitive domain.

Following are the scripts for four vignettes or incidents that were videotaped, the questions based on the vignettes, and some suggested answers.*

VIDEOTAPED VIGNETTES

Vignette A
Incident: Group Process
Site: Nurses' Library
Time: 1 P.M.
Meeting: Weekly meeting of In-service Instructors with Nursing Care
        Coordinators
Cast: 1 In-service Instructor (the designated leader): Jane
     3 Nursing Care Coordinators
        1 from the Obstetric Service: Helen
        1 from the Medical or Surgical Service: Sally
        1 from the Rehabilitation Service: Betty

*This material was originally developed by faculty of the State University of New York Downstate Medical Center College of Nursing in Brooklyn, N.Y., and has been revised by me.

VIDEO

Shot: 3 members seated at table; they have coffee. In-service instructor on one side of table, other members facing her.
Pan: clock 1 P.M.
Sally enters library.

Helen looks at clock behind Jane which shows 1:08, then looks at Jane.

Jane looks at group.

Pan to door. Betty enters and rushes to a seat. Shuffles through some papers and then nods to group.

Betty starts talking quickly.

Pan to clock, 1:40. Betty still talking.

Sally looks to group for support and response.
Helen addresses herself to Jane.

AUDIO

Idle chatter, but none between coordinators and in-service instructor.

Sally – Voice Over: Another meeting! What a waste of time. My main problem is a backache, and it only gets worse when I sit in meetings.

Helen: Can we get started? We've waited long enough.

Jane: I thought we'd wait for Betty. Why don't we wait another two minutes?

Jane: Now that we are all here, let's get started. I would like to remind you all that these meetings are your opportunities to plan educational programs as well as discuss problems in the overall functioning of your units.

Betty: Jasper, Cohen, and Staton have been scheduled for transfer to the Acme Nursing Home for the past five days, and Acme maintains there are no beds available. Dr. Mark said Johnston would go to special services . . . .

Betty: . . . consequently three patients are still occupying space in the hall. How will I implement the new assignment we agreed upon three weeks ago when I have all these other problems?

Sally: It takes me three hours to get on my feet in the morning. You wouldn't believe the pain this disc is giving me. I have to sit in a hot bath to mobilize myself. Coming to work requires all the resources I have. Do you have any thoughts on how I can lessen this back pain?

Helen: I have an urgent problem.

VIDEO	AUDIO
	We have fifteen new cases of staph in the newborn nursery. I have to get an immediate in-service teaching of isolation procedures for my staff.
Pan: Camera on leader who leans back in chair. *Sally and Betty looking at each other.*	*Betty:* Sally, I think you would do well to contact Dr. Sure about your back. He is the best orthopedic surgeon we have on the staff. He seems to take care of all the nurses who have back problems.
Jane looks to group.	*Jane:* Could we get back to the subject?
Helen looks frustrated.	*Helen—Voice over:* What subject? Who can remember what's been going on?

Vignette B
Incident: The Ward Clerk Quits
Site: Nurses' Station, Ward
　　　Clerk's Desk
Time: 8 A.M.
Cast: 1 Registered Nurse: Mrs. Clark
　　　1 Ward Clerk: Ms. Grey

Short pan of entrance to hospital unit. *Close-up of Ms. Grey sitting at desk answering phone. There is a pile of charts at her side. She appears harried and is writing hurriedly.* *Mrs. Clark appears at desk.*	*Mrs. Clark:* I'm Mrs. Clark, a per diem nurse and I will be in charge of the unit today.
Ms. Grey looks up, smiles, says "hi" in an offhand manner and goes back to writing.	*Ms. Grey:* Hi.
	Mrs. Clark: Go to the pharmacy and pick up the A.M. medications.
Ms. Grey looks up with an expression of disbelief and speaks defensively.	*Ms. Grey:* That is not part of my job, Mrs. Clark.
Camera: Close-up of Mrs. Clark's face.	*Mrs. Clark (snappily):* We *are* short of staff today because of the holiday weekend and you'll just have to pitch in.

VIDEO	AUDIO
Camera follows as Mrs. Clark turns back to Ms. Grey. Camera on Ms. Grey's face.	*Ms. Grey (angry and loud):* That's not my job. I'm tired of having all the responsibility around here. No one can do my job and yet I'm expected to do everyone else's.
Camera follows as Ms. Grey stands up and walks around the desk.	*Ms. Grey:* Well, I quit! I'm going to the hospital administrator's office right now to hand in my resignation!
Camera follows as Ms. Grey storms off the unit. Camera shifts to Mrs. Clark, standing there with her mouth open.	

Vignette C
Incident: Whose Case Load?
Site: Visiting Nurse Association Office
Time: 9 A.M., morning conference time
Cast: 1 new Registered Nurse from a baccalaureate program employed in
      the VNA for 2 months: Margo
      1 Registered Nurse who has been on the VNA staff for 5 years: Alma
      1 Supervisor: Miss Samet

Fadein on Margo who is perusing charts on the desk.	*Margo (thinking aloud):* Mrs. James—why am I seeing her today? She and her new baby were fine last week and Mr. Kane's diabetes is well controlled. His urine has been negative for weeks. Wonder why Miss Samet wants me to see these people today. (pause) Mr. Lane and Mrs. Chin sure need visiting, but why do Mrs. Wiley and Mr. Brown? Seems that the supervisor is sure pushing cardiac evaluations and postmastectomy patients this month. (pause) And poor Mr. Comet! He really needs a lot of health teaching with those terrible draining ulcers and his deep depression now that Mrs. Comet is gone.
Camera on Alma entering room with two cups of coffee.	*Alma:* Hi, Margo. Want some coffee?

VIDEO	AUDIO
	Margo: That sounds good.
Alma hands coffee to Margo and remains standing. *Margo uses hand gestures and looks up at Alma.*	
	Margo (sounding frustrated): Say Alma, why does my case load always seem so filled with so many people who really don't need frequent visits? It seems, well, ridiculous to hurry around and see so many patients when I could better use my time spending it with those who really need nursing care.
Alma sips coffee and uses hand gestures.	*Alma (sounding relaxed and confident):* Cool it, you'll soon learn the ropes. Numbers count around here. Who do you think will pay our salaries if we don't see a full case load each day? Besides, these people can always use another visit. Many are lonely.
Margo uses hand gestures, looks up at Alma, frustrated.	*Margo:* Well, I really feel that only three of my seven cases really need me today. I want to spend more time with Mr. Comet especially. What do you think the supervisor will say?
Alma smiles.	*Alma (firmly):* Don't rock the boat! You baccalaureate grads have to hit the real world sooner or later. Take my advice and ease into the system before you try to think for our dear old stonewall supervisor. (pause) Catch you later—I've got work to do.
Alma leaves. Margo focuses on charts for a few seconds. Miss Samet enters, walking rapidly, and stands over Margo.	*Miss Samet (rapidly):* Well, Margo, you're all set with seven cases, aren't you? Let's see if we can get out of the office sooner today.
Miss Samet starts to walk away. *Margo turns around toward her.*	*Margo (hesitantly):* Miss Samet, could I speak with you just a minute?

VIDEO

AUDIO

Miss Samet: Well, make it short, Margo.

Margo: I've been looking over my case load and I feel that Mr. Comet needs more health teaching. (pause)
And he's been so depressed. I feel I must sit down and talk with him and help him to explore his feelings in much greater depth than I've had time to do. If I . . . .

Miss Samet turns toward door to talk to someone offstage.

Miss Samet (impatiently and loudly): It's who, Mildred? Well, tell her I'll call her back—I'm busy. Yes, Margo, go on but hurry it.

Margo (timidly but steadily): I was saying that if I could delay these four cases for today, then I could give more time to Mr. Comet and also Mr. Lane, and Mrs. Chin could use more in-depth teaching. (pause)
The other four patients you gave me for today could be picked up tomorrow.

Miss Samet looks at a few charts. She is not smiling.

Miss Samet (adamantly and firmly): No, Margo. Kane, Brown, and Wiley must be seen today. See James tomorrow if you must, but the others have to be seen.

Margo (pleading): But, Miss Samet . . . .

Miss Samet (firmly): I haven't time to listen now.

Miss Samet leaves.
Fadeout on Margo who looks angry.

Vignette D
Incident: A Change in Method of Assignment
Site: Nurses' Station
Time: 8 A.M., morning report
Cast: 1 Team Leader: Miss Carl
    1 Registered Nurse: Mrs. Zane
    1 Licensed Practical Nurse (no lines)
    1 Nurse's Aide (no lines)

Group seated around team leader who is holding Kardex.

Miss Carl: Mrs. Zane, today you have the same patients you've had

VIDEO	AUDIO
	for the past two days. Mr. Rank in 504, a 70-year-old retired cop who had a cerebrovascular accident, was as cranky as ever last night. He rang his call button all night and soiled his bed three times. There are no changes in his orders.
Mrs. Zane is taking notes on her assignment. She becomes increasingly more irritated as the team leader continues.	You also have Miss Berg in 506, a 26-year-old five-day postop hysterectomy. She was upset and cried most of the night. She was medicated two times for sleep. She'll need a lot of emotional support. And you have Mr. Maxwell in 505, a 36-year-old teacher who has renal calculi. He had quite a bit of pain last night and was medicated one time.
Close-up of Mrs. Zane. *Close-up of team leader listening calmly to Mrs. Zane. Then camera on both.*	*Mrs. Zane (angrily):* I can't possibly take care of those three again! The last two days were bad enough. Mr. Rank needs lots of care with his tube feedings, range-of-motion exercises, turning him every two hours, complete bed bath, and *now* how many times will I have to change his bed because he's incontinent! If I do all that, I can't give any attention to Miss Berg and she *certainly* needs me. Even though Mr. Maxwell doesn't need me to give him a lot of physical care, he doesn't cooperate, and it took me a long time to get him to walk yesterday. This assignment is *much* too heavy. When Mrs. Connell was team leader, she never made us take the same patients every day.
Close-up of Miss Carl.	*Miss Carl (calmly):* Mrs. Zane, by now you should understand what I'm trying to accomplish by instituting continuity of care on this unit. That's why you have the same assignment every day and will have until your patients go home. You know that any problems you have in planning or caring for any of the patients you have can be brought up at team conference.
Fadeout.	

FOLLOWUP QUESTIONS AND ANSWERS ON VIGNETTES*

General Instructions: You will be shown four short videotaped simulations of situations likely to occur in any fairly large agency. Each situation is three or four minutes long and all of them will be shown straight through. The second time you are shown the simulations, select one of them to respond to. Each situation has four essay questions that follow a brief written description of the incident. You will have 40 minutes to answer the questions on one situation.

After a brief recess, you will be shown the videotapes a third time. Select a second situation to which you wish to respond. Again, four essay questions follow the brief written description of the incident and as before, you will have 40 minutes for answering the second set of questions.

In answering the questions related to each incident, you are expected to consider the following variables:

1. Accountability
2. Group dynamics
3. Planned change
4. Priority setting

Questions

Vignette A:

Incident: Group Process

In Hospital X, weekly meetings are held between nursing care coordinators and nursing in-service educators. The purposes of these meetings are to plan in-service programs and to discuss problems relative to the overall functioning of the units. What you have seen is part of one such meeting.

1. As an observer, what 3 problems related to the functioning of of the group can you identify and describe?
2. If you were the group leader, what 3 actions could you take outside of the group that might increase the group's effectiveness?
   Give your rationale for each action.
   What are the expected outcomes of your actions?
3. What are 3 group role behaviors that you might use to facilitate the group's process?
   Give your rationale for each behavior.
   What are the expected outcomes of your behaviors?
4. What data are necessary in order to evaluate the institutional priority of these weekly meetings?

*Final Examination for Nursing 4250, Leadership in the Delivery of Health Care, Spring, 1977.
104

Vignette B:

Incident: The Ward Clerk Quits

A new per diem nurse is placed in charge of a unit on a weekend. She introduces herself to the ward clerk and then says to the clerk, "Go down to the pharmacy and pick up the A.M. medications." The clerk looks up in disbelief and says defensively, "That is not part of my job." After several more words, the ward clerk walks off the unit to hand in her resignation. What you have just seen is part of the incident.

1. What further information is needed to assess the nature of the conflict between the per diem nurse and the ward clerk? How might personal goals conflict with bureaucratic goals in in this situation?

2. Where does the responsibility for patient care lie in this situation? Discuss briefly.

3. What are the factors that contribute to ineffective communication between the concerned individuals? Discuss briefly.

4. How can this conflict be resolved? What kinds of strategies need to be employed by the nurse in order to avert a similar situation from occurring and to promote more harmonious staff functioning?

Vignette C:

Incident: Whose Case Load?

A situation involving conflict between a staff nurse and her supervisor in a Visiting Nurse Association office. The conflict is over priorities regarding which clients should be seen that day. What you have just seen is part of the incident.

1. What strategies could the staff nurse have used to prevent conflict with the supervisor?

2. What strategies can the staff nurse use to resolve this conflict with the supervisor?

3. What effect is the situation as depicted likely to have in terms of accountability for both the supervisor and the staff nurse?

4. If you were the supervisor, how would you change the method of patient assignment so that it would be more effective for both clients and nurses?

Vignette D:

Incident: A Change in Method of Assignment

A new method of daily assignment (assigning the same patients to the same staff) has been introduced by the team leader. The intent of this practice is to promote continuity of patient care. The registered nurse team member objects to her assignment. What you have just seen is part of the incident.

1. What additional information do you need in this situation relative to each of the following:

a. clients
b. team leader
c. team members
d. method of assignment

2. What 5 factors should the team leader have considered in making the assignments to team members?
3. How could you as the team leader have handled the present situation so that the registered nurse team member might have been more receptive to this method of assignment?
4. What strategies could you as the team leader use in order to better effect the change in method of assignment?

Suggested Answers

The answers listed below are to be used as guidelines. Student responses that answer the questions appropriately but differ from the answer suggested may also be acceptable.

The method of scoring used by the faculty was as follows: 25 percent was awarded for each question in one vignette, and each question was granted 1 to 10 points. A perfect total score for one question was 40 points. Two perfect scores of 40 each, or a total score of 80, was then equated to 100; an appropriate conversion table was used for scores below 100.

Vignette A
QUESTION 1
1. Lack of consensus regarding group goals or purposes.
2. Lack of member accountability. Although time is being wasted, no one takes the responsibility for facilitating decision-making or change.
3. Possibility of conflict between the two stated goals or purposes that may be confusing and disruptive to the group.
4. Ineffective leadership.
   a. No effort was made to clarify goals or to refocus group.
   b. No apparent tactics demonstrated for handling the monopolizer.
   c. No response to the expressed problems of the group members.
   d. Laissez-faire style leads to lack of group cohesion.
QUESTION 2
1. Prepare and circulate the agenda in advance in order to encourage preparation for the meeting.
2. Provide leadership in locomotion of the group, e.g., refocus, clarify, tactfully interrupt the monopolizer and relate what she is saying to the group goals, call for a response of the group members regarding consensus.
3. Provide adequate time for the meeting. Try to find out the best time for all of the participants. Begin and end the meeting on time. Indicate the seriousness of the purposes.

4. Carry out measures necessary to bring about desired changes in the coordinators. Seek necessary support from and provide the communication link with leadership and power within the administration. Administrative power is needed behind such efforts.
5. Spend time with group members outside of the meeting, assisting them with their clinical problems and assessing their in-service needs. These actions will help to establish rapport and demonstrate a connection between in-service education and their real clinical problems.

QUESTION 3

The answers should speak to task and maintenance functions but do not have to be labeled as such. Roles must be identified: clarifier, elaborator, coordinator, evaluator, standard setter, refocuser, supporter, harmonizer, gate-keeper, and so on.

QUESTION 4

1. Where did the idea originate? What were the explicit and implicit purposes?
2. What functions does the in-service instructor serve in this institution?
   What status does she have?
3. What are the backgrounds and preparation of the nursing staff for their roles? What are their priorities?
4. What are the nursing service problems at this time? How urgent are they?

Vignette B

QUESTION 1

1. The nurse should know what the responsibilities of the job of ward clerk are and vice versa.
2. How long has the ward clerk worked there?
3. What is the usual practice for getting medications on the weekend?
4. Get to know the staff before making demands of them.
5. Each staff member should know the lines of authority.

QUESTION 2

1. Obviously it is the nurse's responsibility.
2. The philosophy of the organization should reflect that nurses are responsible for patient care.
3. Professional responsibility includes helping staff to work together to give better patient care.
4. What are the implications of the nurse's actions on patient care?

QUESTION 3

1. The style of the nurse: how does she project herself?
2. The effectiveness of the leadership.
3. The status needs of the individuals.
4. The attitudes of the individuals expressed both verbally and behaviorally.
5. The completeness of the assessment as described in Question 1.

QUESTION 4

1. Using resources: who knows what to do, when, and how?
2. Knowing what's involved in the job.
3. Explaining the situation to the clerk, e.g., "There's nothing I can do about it. Would you mind . . . ." Emphasizing the helpful role rather than a subservient one.
4. Investigating other avenues open to her.
5. Sitting down together and deciding what can be done before the situation becomes explosive.

Vignette C

QUESTION 1

1. Assess the situation, e.g., was the timing appropriate, what was the nature of communication? Was the supervisor really involved in problem-solving or in providing alternatives? What are the job descriptions, the roles and responsibilities of the supervisor? What are the policies of the employing agency? How does the supervisor usually react to change? Is there feedback from one's peers?
2. Involve the supervisor in helping the staff nurse to plan care, e.g., "You seem to think I'm slow. Could you suggest some alternatives?"
3. Involve the peer group in the need for change in the method of making out assignments. Get their support first.
4. Offer alternatives when first presenting the situation, not just "I'm seeing four clients."
5. Schedule a specific time, allowing sufficient leeway for discussion.

QUESTION 2

1. Recognize that the strategy used was counterproductive, which also involves awareness of self. Deal with the anger. Talk to her peers.
2. Ask for a conference with enough leeway for discussion.
3. Discuss her perception of the problem with and ask for alternatives from the supervisor.
4. Discuss alternatives with the peer group.

QUESTION 3

1. Agency accountability: standards, National League for Nursing (NLN) accreditation standards, community pressures.
2. Nurse accountability: professional standards, job description, evaluation process, the focus of evaluation, American Nurses' Association (ANA) minimum standards, standards for Public Health Nursing. When should she tell the other clients she will return? How precise was her time assessment? Did she plan carefully or guess? Regarding her time, is overtime a possibility?
3. Supervisor accountability: has accountability changed due to increased education? She knows she could see all clients and give "good" care. How demonstrated and measured?

4. The effect is anxiety for both:

Supervisor—being questioned → Demoralization
Nurse—being boxed in → Apathy

QUESTION 4
1. Assess each nurse's ability, preference, and behavior.
2. Offer constructive feedback.
3. Aim for a balance between variety and consistency of assignment in relation to motivation and productivity of staff.
4. Be more democratic in dealing with professionals.
5. Involve staff nurses in primary planning because it increases motivation for planning and implementing assignments.
6. Be more aware of regularly scheduled meetings. Allow alternatives for quick conferences.
7. Be approachable in terms of communication, phrasing, and content.

Vignette D
QUESTION 1
1. Assignment method.
   a. Present nursing service policy.
   b. Why was it planned?
      Institutional goal ⎫
      Team leader goal   ⎬ to improve quality of care.
      Experimental study ⎭
   c. Who planned this change?
      Hierarchy.
      Team leader decision alone.
      Team members' input.
2. Team leader.
   a. Professional background.
   b. Length and type of experience.
      How long a team member?
      How long a team leader?
      Job description of team leader.
3. Team members.
   a. Length and type of experience.
   b. How long a member of the team?
   c. How long worked with this team leader?
   d. How long worked with other team leaders?
   e. Previous input as to their assignment.
   f. Clients: number and complexity of care.
QUESTION 2
1. Number of patients.
2. Needs of patients.
3. Types of personnel on team and their job descriptions.
4. Number of members on team.
5. Number of each type of personnel on team.

QUESTION 3

1. Reemphasize that the purpose of nursing is to meet patients' needs.
2. Ask the registered nurse to give her reason or rationale as to why she thinks that continuous changing of assignments meets patients' needs.
3. Give your own rationale as to why this method is more apt to meet patients' needs better than the other method.
4. Ask members to try this method and make a comparison, giving the results at the afternoon team conference.
5. Point out that other members of the team are also having the same assignment.
6. Ask the team members if they would like to plan a conference to discuss assignment methods.
7. Reemphasize the purpose of the team, e.g., responsible for groups of patients, working together, willingness to help each other.
8. Suggest to the registered nurse that together you look at what needs to be done.
   a. Help determine patients' needs.
   b. Establish priority of those needs.
   c. Identify where help is needed.

QUESTION 4

1. Plan conferences at a convenient time for total staff participation (all three shifts) so that personnel can analyze the quality of care being given.
2. Personnel should investigate possible methods of assignment, using the literature, the head nurse, the supervisor, in-service education personnel, experts within the institution if possible, and experts from outside the institution.
3. Personnel should compare various methods.
   a. Encourage all members to participate
   b. Acknowledge all contributions.
   c. Weigh the pros and cons of each method, for patients and for members.
4. Utilize informal group structure and focus on informal leaders within the group to encourage the members to implement change.
5. The group should decide how to implement the change.
6. The group should establish the length of the trial period.
7. The group should decide how to review or evaluate, using criteria, and how often it should be done.
8. Determine the changes in implementation as needed and institute change.
9. The team should report as to the effectiveness of the change to the head nurse and supervisor (reward system).

REFERENCES

1. Berger, M. M. (Ed.) *Videotape Techniques in Psychiatric Training and Treatment.* New York: Brunner/Mazel, 1970.
2. Boyd, J. L., Jr., and Shimberg, B. *Handbook of Performance Testing.* Princeton, N.J.: Educational Testing Service, 1971.
3. Crosby, M. H. Teaching strategies: A microteaching project for nurses in Virginia. *Nurs. Res.* 26:144, 1977.
4. de Tornyay, R. Instructional technology and nursing education. *J. Nurs. Educ.* 9:3, 1970.
5. Dietrich, B. J., and Merrill, I. R. Television in health sciences education: Camera placement. *Nurs. Res.* 13:217, 1964.
6. Eggert, L. L. Challenge exam in interpersonal skills. *Nurs. Outlook* 23:707, 1975.
7. Frejlach, G., and Corcoran, S. Measuring clinical performance. *Nurs. Outlook* 19: 270, 1971.
8. Griffin, G. J., Kinsinger, R. E., and Pitman, A. J. Clinical nursing instruction and closed circuit TV. *Nurs. Res.* 13:196, 1964.
9. Griffin, G. J., Kinsinger, R., Pitman, A., and Kessler, E. New dimensions for the improvement of critical nursing. *Nurs. Res.* 15:292, 1966.
10. Hess, J. W. A comparison of methods for evaluating medical student skill in relating to patients. *J. Med. Educ.* 44:934, 1969.
11. Hoose, D. C. A model for a nursing media center. *Nurs. Outlook* 24:104, 1976.
12. Koch, H. B. Television in nursing education. *J. Nurs. Educ.* 7:37, 1968.
13. Koch, H. B. Autotutorial instruction. *Nurs. Outlook* 23:619, 1975.
14. Koch, H. B. Film or television? *Nurs. Outlook* 23:489, 1975.
15. Koch, H. B. Production and technical standards. *Nurs. Outlook* 23:287, 1975.
16. Koch, H. B. Satellites and video discs. *Nurs. Outlook* 23:743, 1975.
17. Lange, C. M. *Autotutorial Techniques in Nursing Education.* Englewood Cliffs, N.J.: Prentice-Hall, 1972.
18. Lange, C. M. Matching media to learning styles. *Nurs. Outlook* 25:18, 1977.
19. Lange, C. M. Using media in evaluation. *Nurs. Outlook* 25:241, 1977.
20. Murray, M. *The Videotape Book.* New York: Bantam Books, 1975.
21. Preparing a teleclass: A case study. *Nurs. Outlook* 23:681, 1975.
22. Quiring, J. The autotutorial approach: Effect of timing of videotape feedback on sophomore nursing students' achievement of skill in giving subcutaneous injections. *Nurs. Res.* 21:332, 1972.
23. Rogers, S. Testing the RN student's skills. *Nurs. Outlook* 24:446, 1976.
24. Sealy, S. Videosociology students utilize TV technology . . . to put social patterns in perspective. *Hunter News* 6:4, 1976.
25. Smith Holland, J. A. Videotaping clinical experience. *Nurs. Outlook* 25:337, 1977.
26. Smyth, K., and McMahon, J. A workshop approach to continuing education. *Nurs. Educator* 1:16, 1976.
27. Sullivan, J. A., et al. Video mediated self-cognition and the Amidon-Flanders interaction analysis model in the training of nurse practitioners' history taking skills. *J. Nurs. Educ.* 14:39, 1975.
28. Taylor, C. B. To videotape or not to videotape. *Audiovisual Instruct.* 22:33, 1977.
29. Thompson, M. L., Chattin, J. A., and Balestrieri, M. Use of instructional television: A shared program. *J. Am. Dietet. Assoc.* 67:573, 1975.

30. Turner, E. V., Helper, M., Kriska, S., Singer, S., and Ruma, S.   Evaluating clinical skills of students in pediatrics. *J. Med. Educ.* 47:959, 1972.
31. Watts, M. W., Jr.   Behavior modeling and self-devaluation with video self-confrontation. *J. Educ. Psychol.* 64:212, 1973.

6. Written Simulations

The criticisms levelled against paper-and-pencil multiple-choice questions are legend. Among the complaints offered is that the level of cognition tested is low. If one examines the tests developed by faculty in many schools of nursing, the majority of questions are indeed at the lower levels of the cognitive domain. It is not uncommon to find an inordinate percentage of items that test definitions, terms, and related minutiae. Do not assume from this statement that all such questions are unimportant. Their importance or unimportance depends on many things and one of them is certainly the level of the student. In many early courses in nursing, practical and registered nurse courses, as well as in the health-related professions, students do need to know terminology and facts. It is when questions aimed at the recall of isolated facts constitute the bulk of an examination given close to graduation, and when faculty claim such questions assess the nurse's ability to function as a graduate, that I get concerned. We can ask ourselves if it really makes a difference in patient care if a nursing student knows who wrote what article or what the name of an instrument is, especially one that is only rarely used!

The complaint that questions test very little of importance is relatively easy to remedy by specifically designing questions to assess higher levels of cognition, for example, analysis; the test contained in Chapter 3 includes such questions. An approach that facilitates writing questions at the higher levels of the cognitive domain is to base them on behavioral objectives (this presupposes that the objectives are more than of the "knows," "lists," "describes" category.) If the objectives are clearly stated and include only one discrete behavior, test questions directly related to them are more likely to result. The key word is *behavior*. An objective that states "Analyzes the effects of an adaptation in a nursing procedure" can lead to the development of a number of questions assessing that objective. All that has to be decided is the nursing procedure, the condition or disease that the patient has, and the modification that is to be tested.

More germane to the issue at hand, however, is the complaint that problem-solving skills, clinical judgment in nursing, and decision-making ability (without the choices being given in the options) are not being adequately assessed. It is primarily for this reason that the uses of simulations in nursing have been explored.

In order to have a common frame of reference, a definition of simulation is needed. Surprisingly, that task was not easily accomplished. Two dictionaries were not very useful, nor were the majority of references. It would appear that most authors assume that everyone knows what is meant by the term, which is perhaps justifiable since who isn't familiar with the simulations of the astronauts' walk and ride on the moon. In the review of the literature, however, it was apparent that not all used the term in the same way. Although Clark's [13, p. 4] definition (credit is given to D. A. Sleet)—"A simulation creates an experiential situation which mimics processes or conditions that occur in the real world"—is the best and most concise, it is not complete. Much greater detail is given by Fitzpatrick and Morrison [21] and by McGuire and her colleagues [46] in their superb book on written simulations. Those wishing more information on the development of written simulations should consult those works, particularly the latter.

Games and gaming strategies have been included by some authors under the umbrella of simulation. Hayman [29] states that "Games may be used to present information, exercise skill, assess performance, and provide substitute or simulated situations." Also mentioned is the fact that they "mirror some aspect of reality," and can be used in interpersonal relation situations and in mock patient-care units. Because of my own philosophy I would choose not to include games in any evaluation program to assess the nurse's ability to give patient care. Learning to be a nurse is serious business and although games can be used effectively in teaching and as part of formative evaluation (diagnostic testing), I would prefer that games per se not be used in the summative evaluation of nursing competence.

The purpose of simulation exercises, according to Lange [36], is to "present learning experiences specifically designed to represent actual problems by providing the learner with the essential aspects of the real situation without its hazards, costs, or time limitations." With minor revisions, this statement of purpose could be applied to simulations developed for use in testing.

For use in learning situations, Lange's statement provides direction to faculty members interested in designing and using simulations in their classes. With a little imagination, one could design simulations to take the place of patient-care situations hard to come by. A constant traffic of health personnel in the room of a patient with an esoteric condition is an all too common problem in hospitals, especially large medical centers. If a simulation of that situation could be designed, how beneficial it would be for the real patient. The same behaviors that can be practiced and learned via simulations are also testable in simulations: demonstrating the ability to gather data, interpreting data, setting priorities, making clinical nursing judgments, using a variety of resources, taking appropriate action, altering a situation by intervention, evaluating the effects of the intervention, and revising the plan of care based on the evaluation.

TYPES OF SIMULATION

Although most of the literature deals with written simulations, there are other kinds, as well as combinations of them, in use.* Oral simulations based on role-playing have been used both in testing and in teaching. One of the main differences between role-playing and oral simulations is that

---

*Although computer simulations exist for the purpose of teaching, testing, and research, they have not been included. To go into detail about the development of a simulation test utilizing a computer would have required time and equipment above and beyond the limits of this book. However, some of the maxims applicable to written simulations are also appropriate for computer simulations.

the former typically is spontaneous although with perhaps some guidelines as to the direction the situation is to go, while the latter is generally
more specific. With an oral simulation, there may be a script for the actors
to follow or the vignette may be developed in sufficient detail to allow the
actors to present the same situation again and again.

Using simulated or programmed patients, so aptly discussed and utilized
by Barrows [6], is basically an extension of an oral simulation. Persons,
not necessarily professional or even amateur actors, are hired to portray
real patients. They are provided with a detailed script, which Barrows
calls a protocol (the example he gives looks like most patient histories one
is likely to see in any hospital in a grand rounds presentation, clinical
conference, or in any medical journal), and are given the opportunity to
rehearse until they can truly simulate a real patient and can do so over and
over again with countless medical students. Additional simulations can be
added as appropriate to the situation by presenting, for example, laboratory reports, X-ray films, electroencephalogram (EEG) or electrocardio-
gram (EKG) readings. All simulations can be tested with latent-image,
conventional multiple-choice, or computer-linked examinations. The
student's performance is videotaped. Barrows includes a checklist for
observing and rating the student and a report that is submitted by the
simulated patient.

Another type of simulation is a mock-up of a real environment and
involves training or testing performance, or both. Fitzpatrick and Morrison
[21] discuss simulations in relation to performance and product evaluation and include the following kinds of tests: situational, in-basket, work-
sample, and diagnostic problem-solving. Examples of performance tests
they cite include those used in stenography, language, automobile operation, art, music, industrial arts, agriculture, and sports and physical fitness.
Since the application of performance tests utilizing the simulation concept
has great relevance to nursing, Chapter 7 is devoted to further exploration
and discussion of mock clinical settings and gives an example of a performance test in such a setting.

The third category of simulations—written simulations—is by far the
most publicized and is more widely used in medicine and nursing than are
oral or performance simulations. Although I am tempted to say that written simulations are more highly developed than are the other types, it
would not be true. Some of the performance simulations or actual simulators are so sophisticated and technologically advanced (and, as a result, so
prohibitive financially) that written simulations seem in comparison like
child's play.

As currently developed, the majority of written simulations are of the
sequential type and use either a linear or branching mode; several branching techniques have been employed. They require the examinee to choose
from an almost unlimited number of responses (limited only by the
creativity of the test developer and by plausibility of the choices) and
in the case of multiple routes, to choose the safest, most efficient, economical, and accurate route, along with whatever else the examinee is

directed to do. The chief purported advantage of the branching method is that since different persons may arrive at successful solutions to a problem in different ways, alternate pathways must be provided.

A highly recommended reference source for the novice on simulation and gaming is a chapter by Paul Twelker [54] in the book *The Guide to Simulation Games For Education and Training*. Included in his chapter is a guide to the literature in the form of an annotated bibliography, a list of journals and newsletters geared to the topic, professional organizations that are interested in the subject, either as their major focus or as one of several, and groups that are actively involved in developing simulations and games.

WHY USE SIMULATIONS?

The most obvious answer to the question of why simulations should be used for testing purposes is that they have face validity, or as applied to simulations, fidelity. Since they are purposely designed to represent reality, students find them more relevant than conventional multiple-choice questions and do get involved. (In defense of multiple-choice questions, however, they too can be made more acceptable if they are built around the needs of a patient.) Perhaps there would be less resistance to tests on the part of students if tests looked more like the real world.

A second reason for using simulations is that the tests currently in use in most schools do not assess the ability of students to make decisions, solve problems, use judgment in deciding on a course of action, and the like. This problem alone is a major justification for the development and use of simulations.

Another reason for their use is that patient situations are typically more complex than the usual multiple-choice examination questions would indicate. In writing multiple-choice questions, one strives for the inclusion of only essential content, for conciseness along with clarity, and for the avoidance of unintentional clues. In any simulation the surround is important (especially in performance tests), and directions are given to include some extraneous material since real patients do give information that is irrelevant. In general, only one aspect of content is tested in a multiple-choice question; in written simulations, on the other hand, many aspects are included because the student must sift out the relevant from the irrelevant in a patient who may have a multi-faceted problem. Hayman [29] lends support to this latter statement by saying "Some simulations over-simplify the real situation. They include only a limited number of variables that influence the problem, whereas real-life situations are much more complex."

WHEN TO USE SIMULATIONS

The question of when to use simulations is in part linked to the why of their use. When one needs to assess those abilities, such as decision-making listed above, that are not measurable by other means, for example, by multiple-choice questions, simulations may be the solution. Simulations can also be used for diagnosing students' areas of strengths and weaknesses and if and in what areas assistance is needed (formative evaluation). They can also be used at the end of a unit or course or at a time close to graduation (summative evaluation). They are certainly useful for self-evaluation. And because immediate feedback is possible, they offer much potential in continuing education programs. With issues of relicensure and recertification constantly on the horizon, simulations seem a logical, theoretically sound way to go.

HOW SIMULATIONS HAVE BEEN USED

Simulations and games as we know them have been used in industry, business, and education for better than a decade. Although not always called simulations, they had some of the characteristics of such tools. One widely discussed situational test simulates an administrator's job and is called an in-basket test. Developed by Frederiksen and his colleagues [23], the technique has been adapted by others for use with, for example, school principals and the police force [21].

In another application of simulation, Flagle [22] describes the use of a simulation system in the study and administration of health services. The definition he offers is different in some ways from those of others. He says that "it is a model-building technique for forecasting how systems, as yet unbuilt, will behave. It is an adjunct of the decision-making process, a way of creating and testing alternative systems or approaches to problem solving." Based on that definition, the possibilities for adaptation of his model seem infinite.

Recently a school brochure listed a course called "The City Game" that is described as follows:

Simulation of urban development of a rural area. Game players will buy and sell real estate, invest in business and housing, and manage municipal affairs. They seek practical ways out of city problems as they see these troubles develop in simulation [30].

Without a doubt there are similar offerings in many other colleges and universities, and the likelihood of new offerings can be anticipated. Simulations and games are still developmentally mere babes, with the best yet to come.

Medicine appears to have taken the giant step in the development and use of simulation techniques for assessing clinical competence. The following descriptions of such developments and use in medicine are only a representative sample—no attempt was made to be exhaustive.

Patient-management problems have been used in Part III of the National Board of Medical Examiner's certification examination since 1961 [33, p. 43]. These programmed tests, initially called tab tests, are among the types of tests designed to assess the problem-solving abilities of physicians, the ultimate purpose of Part III. Patient-management problems are also used in the National Board's physician's assistant examination, and in their pediatric nurse practitioner and associate examination. A special project of the National Board has been the development of a Comprehensive Qualifying Examination to determine the readiness of physicians for graduate medical education. One part of that study involves the comparison of various methods of presenting patient-management problems [48, p. 29]. An excellent sample of patient-management problems used in the National Board examinations is given in Dr. Hubbard's book, *Measuring Medical Education* [33], which discusses the examinations and the procedures utilized by the National Board.

The National Board, however, has not limited itself to patient-management problems; it has been developing branching clinical simulations and computer-based simulations [48, p. 26]. Another of their studies entails not only paper-and-pencil branching simulations, but audiovisual simulations and programmed patients. The data generated from this latter study, presently being analyzed, should be illuminating because of the comparison of the three types of simulation techniques [48, p. 25].

Although not the primary purpose of the study, paper-and-pencil clinical simulations were utilized in a study by McCarthy [39, p. 263]. He was interested in the performance of medical students on tests that provided visual cues as compared with an oral free-response format. The simulation examination was of the erasure type, in which information is provided when the appropriate space is erased. In his discussion of the results, McCarthy states:

... the printed erasure problem appears to constitute a significant advance in the evaluation of clinical competence. It enables the examinee to perform a total evaluation of a clinical problem and it permits this to happen in the sequential fashion utilized by the practicing physician [39, p. 266].

Goran and others [25, p. 171] in their study of the validity of patient-management problems (PMP) included in their discussion the fact that:

... cueing may artificially inflate scoring on PMP's as much as 25 percent. In a PMP the examinee is asked to select from a list of options the data he would like to elicit. It is not possible to ascertain whether the examinee does, in fact, have knowledge of the pertinent questions [25, p. 176].

According to the author, the point that performance on the patient-management test problem was better for the average physician than was his performance in actual practice further illustrates the effect of cueing.

Because of conflicting results obtained by other researchers regarding what factors underlie performance on patient-management problems, Juul and her colleagues [34] at the University of Illinois Medical Center undertook to study the problem further. At issue was whether the patient-management problems measured a general skill in medical problem-solving or whether separate and distinct skills were involved, namely information-gathering and decision-making. Among the findings in earlier studies was that medical problem-solving was content-specific and that information-gathering was a general ability [34, p. 2].

In Juul's study, the results suggested that data-gathering and management factors were not independent. Further, the authors state:

It seems likely that appropriate management of a patient is to a certain extent dependent on the adequacy of the data base developed from the history, physical, and diagnostic procedures. However, an examinee might ask all the right questions but not be able to integrate the information to arrive at an appropriate resolution to the problem, or he might arrive at the appropriate resolution from a sketchy data base [34, p. 7].

This statement has implications in a number of situations. Too often a student is given credit, for example, for applying principles in a multiple-choice test question, when in fact the correct answer could be arrived at in several other ways: recall of what she saw, recall of what an instructor said, or all of the options in the question dealt with the application of principles. The study also included advice to include a wide sample of patient-management problems, something that test constructors attempt to do in developing a test's table of specifications (test blueprint).

In one stage of a multiphasic project, McGuire and her colleagues [40, p. 267] studied the oral examination used to assess the clinical competence of physicians. Included in the investigation were observer training sessions that included how to use the form for recording observations and then the use of those forms with two simulated oral examinations. It should be obvious that since subjectivity has been a major disadvantage in the use of such examinations, this phase of the study was aimed at minimizing that problem. Inter-rater reliability was concurrently determined by using pairs of experienced examiners. An interesting finding, though not unexpected, was that "nearly 70 percent of the questions [asked by the examiners] were judged to require predominantly only the recall of information [40, p. 269]."

The magnitude of this study, the results, and the implications have been minimized here but one widely disseminated conclusion of this part of the project led to a healthy skepticism about the use of the oral examination not only for assessing the clinical competence of physicians but in other fields as well. (See also the article by Levine and McGuire [38] on the validity and reliability of oral examinations.)

The third stage of the study, concerned with developing new methods for evaluating clinical competence, led to the development of, among others, a well-defined oral simulation involving role-playing and the use of a checklist that included content, attitude, and performance criteria [42]. A demonstration of a crisis situation centered around a 2-year-old boy who had swallowed aspirin was presented at the 1972 National Council of Measurement in Education annual conference in Chicago by staff of the Center for Educational Development, University of Illinois College of

Medicine. The checklist developed for use with that simulation was distributed and included, under content, criteria questions such as "How is
he breathing?" and "Does family have syrup of ipecac at home?" Under
the attitudinal criteria was the statement "Acted toward the family as if:"
which was to be rated on a scale of 1 to 5, with the extremes representing
criticizing and supporting behaviors; three others were also included. The
performance criteria listed only two, one of which was "Gave family an
organized set of doctor's instructions and required the family to repeat
them back [11]."

I have neither seen nor heard about any further developments nor uses
of these oral simulations since a 1972 article [35, p. 789], but there is a
place for them, if not in evaluation, certainly in teaching.

The use of simulated patients in the 1970 Certification Examination of
the College of Family Physicians of Canada presents a different approach
to the assessment of physicians' skills [35, p. 789]. In addition to the
typical written examinations, both multiple-choice and patient-management problems, the examination included an oral examination composed
of three parts: (1) a formal oral, (2) a role-playing patient-management
problem, and (3) a simulated office oral [35, p. 789]. This last part of
the examination consisted of actors and actresses who had been "programmed" to play the roles of patients with problems likely to be seen in
the office of a family practitioner. Each of the patient protocols was
standardized to the extent deemed necessary so that each candidate was
presented with essentially the same patient. Every candidate interviewed
three such simulated patients in a predetermined time limit (12 minutes
for each) and was scored simultaneously by two observers who had previously been briefed in the use of the scoring method. Of the five performance factors scored in the simulated office oral examination, the one
given the greatest weight was attitudinal skills [35, p. 791].

The interest in programmed patients undoubtedly led Barrows [6] to
expand his earlier work [3-5], upon which the simulated office oral was
based, to address the many questions that arose from use of the technique
and to discuss in more depth aspects previously treated rather superficially.
For those interested in simulated patients, Barrows' book is highly recommended.

The assessment of the kinds of skills necessary for physicians to diagnose
and relate effectively to patients and others is to be initiated in pre-
medical entrance examinations, according to a recent release from the
Educational Testing Service [14]. The consortium of 13 medical schools
in collaboration with the National Board of Medical Examiners and under
the direction of the Educational Testing Service will be developing simulation tools to assess those activities that are essential for the competent
physician. The two aspects of the project that are of primary concern in
relation to physician performance are diagnostic problem-solving, in particular, clinical problems, and the assessment of interpersonal skills.

Although simulations and simulation games have been used in business
and industry, at universities, and in medicine for some time, their use in

nursing is a relatively recent occurrence. Clark [13, p. 9] says that simulation gaming is in its infancy but that it offers great potential for teaching in nursing, particularly when a change in attitude is desired. She defines simulation games as follows: "The elements in a simulation game are patterned to simulate aspects of the real world, but are structured in a game format with rules, goals, activities, constraints, and payoffs [13, p. 4]."

In her book Bevis [9] devotes several pages to a discussion of games and simulations in relation to learning strategies. Among the situations in which simulations and simulation games are advocated is one in which "the behavior to be learned is hazardous to life or potentially places people in unsafe, uncomfortable, or unhealthy situations."

Neither of these nurse-authors mentions the use of simulations in evaluation but then both were concerned with the teaching aspects of simulations. Nevertheless, the potential is there, waiting to be explored. What follows is an overview of simulation techniques in nursing—both in teaching and evaluation—some of them in use for some time, with special emphasis on written tests.

Use of Simulations in Nursing

Simulations have been used in teaching nursing in a variety of ways and in many different content areas. To satisfy the expressed needs of students in a baccalaureate nursing program for observing a community health nurse making a home visit, films were made of three different situations involving actual patients of qualified community health nurses. These films, part of the instructional package developed by faculty for the course, were used as the basis for discussion. Role-playing as a result of the instructor's question, "How would you have done it?" was seen as a possible extension of the simulation. Another question, "What would you have written if you were preparing the record?" [49] could either be answered orally or the students could be asked to actually write their own version for the patient's record.

Adaptation of this method for evaluation purposes would be relatively simple. As with other methods that are designed for teaching purposes and converted for use in assessment, the method could be used but not the same content. If the content has been specifically taught or discussed at great length in class, when the instrument is used for assessing that content what one usually assesses is memory, at best simple recall. In other words, comparable simulations would have to be developed especially for the purpose of evaluation. The students would then be familiar with the format; and, assuming that the questions are well developed, they could be used to get at knowledge at the higher levels of the cognitive domain. This kind of instrument would be especially useful to get at the level of synthesis.

A multi-media instructional simulation system was developed by faculty in a school of nursing to allow students to practice assessing patient needs [15]. Although it was designed for teaching purposes, the authors state that the system could be used for evaluative purposes. Not stated, however, is the fact that if the system as described is used for teaching purposes, it should probably not be used with the same students for evaluation purposes since it would probably be assessing only memory. However, if sufficient time has elapsed between two administrations, it may provide useful information.

This system can be scored in the same fashion as de Tornyay's test (see p. 123) [17]. Unlike de Tornyay's test, the written portions of the system were produced on reusable booklets with easily removed gummed labels in place of the opaque overlays, a purportedly less expensive method.

The use of visual media with the written simulation seems to have merit since the problem of ambiguity is likely to be diminished. In addition, the adage, "One picture is worth a thousand words," seems appropriate since the use of a visual aid may well cut down on the amount of text to be read. Too often extraneous information is included in the written patient situation and although it may make for interesting reading, it is unnecessary in light of the questions that follow and may in fact be misleading or confusing.

Curtis and Rothert [15] state that other multi-media simulations are planned but as of this writing, I have not seen any reports of their development.

It appears from a review of the literature that the first simulation test in the form of a patient-management problem in nursing was done by McIntyre and her colleagues [47, p. 429] in 1966 and reported in 1972. Designed to evaluate the decision-making abilities of nursing students as they progressed through the then-experimental curriculum, the simulation test was patterned after McGuire and Babbott's model [43] for evaluating comparable abilities in medical students. The content of the simulation test was validated by subject matter experts. Some information also is given about the reliability of the instrument.

The situation developed for this study followed a patient from the time he arrived in the hospital emergency room through his discharge and return to home and community. The patient apparently had a neurological problem since, in the discussion of the test development, specialists in this area validated test content [47, p. 430]. The test consisted of 81 items in two sections, a free response part and a controlled response part that "were classified into five kinds of nursing activities: data-gathering actions, 23; patient care actions, 25; communications, 18; environmental management, 9; professional referrals, 5. One item was related to recording." The report also gives a breakdown of the behavioral responses and the items in each section as well as a sample of each type of item. The opaque overlay procedure used by other test developers was not used for this test, according to the authors, because of time and cost factors. Instead, information was contained in sealed envelopes that were numbered to match the question or action selected.

What was particularly interesting about this project was the extensive scoring system that was developed. In addition to using the one developed by Williamson [47, p. 432; 55] that provided three different indexes—an efficiency index, a proficiency index, and a competency index—four other scores were derived. The second one, used with the controlled response items, was essentially one of rank ordering of item choices with a numerical value assigned to each item. The third score was derived from classifying the controlled response items into one of three categories: (1) required, (2) helpful but not essential, and (3) contraindicated. The fourth score, the major one in terms of evaluating the experimental curriculum, was obtained by classifying the controlled response items according to the level of decision-making involved—from simple recall of information with basically no interpretation of data to simple interpretation of data with the application of a single principle or combination of principles in a typical problem to the more complex level. This particular classification method was utilized by McGuire in an earlier work. The fifth score involved the classification of both controlled response and free response items according to their risk dimension and their value in terms of nursing action and expected outcome. The majority of items were classified as high value and low risk, an anticipated result.

The authors [47, p. 435] conclude with the hope that this type of evaluation tool will be used as a model for the development of others, since the tool does provide information that is especially useful in assessing the clinical competence of nursing students.

One of the earliest simulations in the form of a patient-management problem in nursing was done by de Tornyay [16] and reported in the spring of 1968. More detail about the development of that test and an illustrative example were published later in that same year [17]. The test was designed after the model of McGuire and Babbott's [43] simulated, branched patient-care problem that had been created to assess the problem-solving abilities of medical students.

In addition to making decisions about actions that warranted priority, the nursing student had to make other decisions relative to appropriate interventions or what information it was necessary to obtain. Once that action was taken or the information requested was obtained by erasing the opaque overlay adjoining it, the student then had to decide what the next step should be. Since in this particular format the sequence was scrambled, the student was not given any clues by the arrangement of choices—a decided advantage; otherwise one might be testing the student's ability to take the test rather than the subject matter contained therein, or in this case, the student's problem-solving ability.

Although some simulated tests contain only approved regimens or at least alternatives that would not be harmful, this test also includes choices that would be contraindicated. Such an approach allows for discriminating the borderline student in relation to safety, as well as identifying content inadequately mastered by those students missing the item(s).

The scoring procedure used was a modification of one developed by Williamson [55] (see above).

In the discussion of the validity of the test, it was gratifying to see that content validity was established. The review of early forms of the test by content experts and the documentation of all alternatives in current reference books were specifically cited as being included in the validation process. Reliability coefficients are also reported. Unfortunately these coefficients are rather low.

In addition to its use for the purpose for which it was designed, the use of this simulated test of problem-solving abilities is recommended by the author as an effective teaching tool, allowing the student to make mistakes in a simulated clinical setting. This safeguards the real patient.

A paper-and-pencil simulation test was developed by Gover [26] to measure the difference in problem-solving proficiency between graduates of technical nursing programs (diploma and associate degree) with those of professional nursing programs (baccalaureate). The Nursing Performance Simulation Instrument (NPSI) consists of four simulations containing 126 items and includes representation from the various clinical areas as well as the life cycle. Gover designed the test so that it would reflect typical situations a staff nurse would be likely to meet in the course of her professional experience.

The simulations become increasingly complex as additional information is presented as the situations progress. As contrasted with most paper-and-pencil tests, which focus on the needs of one patient and perhaps his family, this simulation examination presents six patients at the outset with an additional one added toward the end of the test. The format is quite different from most paper-and-pencil tests but seems suited to the intended purpose. Included in the decisions that need to be made are those that deal with priorities (both immediate and those that can be postponed temporarily), role functions, forced-choice actions, referrals, and patient-care assignments to team members; one section involves answering items that deal with some of the knowledge needed to make those decisions.

Two reliability coefficients are reported for the NPSI. The test-retest reliability correlation coefficient was .63 and the Spearman-Brown odd-even correlation coefficient was .58 [26, p. 12]. Of the 126 items in the NPSI, only 53 discriminated the high-scoring nursing educators from the low-scoring nursing educators and are included in the revised version of the NPSI [26, p. 29].

A simulation test was developed by faculty in a school of nursing to assess just prior to graduation their students' decision-making ability in clinical situations [52, p. 458]. Both associate degree and baccalaureate nursing students were included in the study. Situations likely to be encountered in the practice of nursing were developed in the areas of medical-surgical nursing, maternal-child nursing, pediatric nursing, and psychiatric nursing. Each of the four situations contained from three to six episodes and used the branching approach rather than a serial (linear) one. The approach used was justified by faculty because "in clinical situations, different actions usually lead to different outcomes [52, p. 459]." The computer was used as the vehicle for administering the test because, according to Sumida, "it would have been very difficult, if not impossible, to use the standard pencil-and-paper examination format for a branching progression test design [52, p. 459]."

The four categories around which items were developed were observation, communication, manipulation, and cooperation, with each category broken down further. Responses were ordered along a three-point continuum from good to better to best. This ordering of choices differs from most other tests in which were included options that were either detrimental to the patient or were neutral in effect.

Although the situations were developed around the 54 behaviors (previously identified in the nursing program) expected of nursing students at the completion of their educational program, there was not a question for each behavior. Rather, "each response demonstrated one or more of the behaviors from the 54-item list, and it was possible to tally the total number achieved by each student [52, p. 460]."

Among the revisions the author suggests for the future use of this test is the substitution of videotaped clinical situations in place of the written simulations. In addition, the use of the computer simulation test is seen as a potential challenge examination for registered nurse students in a baccalaureate nursing program.

Another written simulation test used to assess clinical judgment in nursing patterned after McGuire's tool was constructed by Dincher and Stidger [18, p. 280]. The patient about whom the simulation was written had had an abdominoperineal resection with a colostomy the day before, performed because the patient had cancer of the sigmoid and rectum [18, p. 281]. The test was developed around the patient's immediate care and later sought to arrive at a nursing diagnosis by investigating in-depth the previously chosen actions.

The latent-image method was used to reveal the information sought by the examinee by applying a developer pen (a chemical is the magic ingredient). The authors suggest this technique should be done commercially rather than within the institution.

Critical-care nurses and associate degree nursing faculty served as both contributors and judges, thereby addressing the instrument's content validity. Also discussed are construct and concurrent validity, which involved ranking the students in order of proficiency in clinical performance and in test performance and then correlating those ranks using Spearman's rho [18, p. 284].

A great deal of information about reliability is presented for all three scores—an adaptation of the same three used by Williamson (see p. 123) [55]. It was not surprising to find the reliability coefficients low in light of the small sample size, eleven.

The sample of actions initially given made me wary of the worth of the entire test because of the overlap of actions, a point made later when the test was critiqued by the panel of experts [18, p. 284]. For example, "observe the patient" and "check the vital signs" can both be done while "visit[ing] the patient," although the students were instructed to choose only one of them. In spite of these and other limitations expressed by the authors about the experimental simulation instrument, they suggest the applicability of the instrument in a great many situations, including the State Board Test Pool licensing examinations. I, for one, would need more proof of the instrument's worth to justify making such a claim.

PREPARING A WRITTEN SIMULATION

The topic of developing a written simulation is dealt with so completely by McGuire and her colleagues [46] in the definitive work on that subject, *Construction and Use of Written Simulations,* that it would be presumptuous of me to attempt any further directives. This volume should be studied prior to embarking on this most challenging venture. As a test constructor, however, I want to mention some precepts that are as relevant to the development of simulations as they are to other kinds of paper-and-pencil tests.

1. The identification of content and objectives in a test blueprint or table of specifications (see pages 25 and 32 in Chap. 3 for examples of such a blueprint) should facilitate isolation of those facets most adaptable to the written simulation format. Since it is unlikely at the outset of developing written simulations that one would attempt an entire examination composed of such simulations, it may be that only some parts of the test blueprint will be reflected in simulation exercises with the bulk of the examination being made up of other kinds of questions. In other words, a test blueprint is not necessary for each simulation, but specific behavioral objectives upon which the simulation is developed are essential. As skill in writing simulations is acquired, a more representative sample of content from the blueprint will be possible.
2. Since familiarity with the technique of written simulations will be limited for many examinees, explicit instructions will be necessary. A short practice exercise will be useful in making examinees feel more comfortable with the format. Also included in the introduction should be information about time limits (one would hope that in nursing the test would be one of power rather than of speed, and that examinees are given sufficient time to attempt to answer all questions) and a simple explanation of the scoring procedure to be used.
3. If displays or other material such as charts, graphs, slides, tape recordings, and the like are to be used with the written simulation, they need to be obtained and checked carefully to make sure that they go with the simulation. For example, a record of vital signs for an infant would be inappropriate for a school-age child. (This latter statement presupposes that the task involved does not necessitate identification of the fact that the vital signs are inappropriate!) If presentation of the display next to the actions that pertain to it are likely to provide unintentional clues to that action, consideration should be given to organizing all

such media in a separate section, although obviously directions will need to be given to the examinee as to where the desired information can be found. Typically all such pictorial displays are given at the end of the simulation.

4. After the simulation has had a dry run or two from your colleagues (expert in the appropriate subject matter) to further polish the exercise and eliminate any sources of ambiguity, the instrument should be administered experimentally to an appropriate sample. As with any paper-and-pencil test, following each tryout revisions should be made based on the students' reactions to and comments on the simulation, and least important in this instance, the data. Since conventional measures of reliability and validity are not applicable to written simulations [46], it is essential that the resulting instrument be as highly refined as possible in order to make any judgments about what students are able to do based on the scores obtained on the simulation.

SCORING A WRITTEN SIMULATION

The majority of scoring methods in use have been based on the work of Williamson [55] and provide an index of the examinee's efficiency, proficiency, and competency. McGuire and her colleagues [46] use the three scores just mentioned and add two others, errors of omission and errors of commission. In addition, they clarify the matter of assigning weights to each of the options and offer both a classification system for the five types of options (ranging from essential to do to essential to avoid) and the numerical weights assigned to options in a nine-level classification system. Formulas for calculating each of the scores are lucidly presented.

Although optical scanners can be used to score written simulations, most of them at this time are not developed to the point of being able to handle the specially designed answer sheets. As a result, computer-scoring or hand-scoring is recommended. If computer services are available to you, by all means consult with the specialists in that area. If they are not, obviously you will need to prepare an answer key for hand-scoring. McGuire and associates [46] provide a form for self-scoring that would be useful to you. And there may be times when you want your students to correct their own examinations. Hand calculators certainly facilitate the scoring procedure.

A SAMPLE WRITTEN SIMULATION

What follows is a portion of a simulation exercise that involves an infant brought to the Well Child Clinic for routine health supervision. It could be included in a course in pediatric nursing or that portion of a course concerned with well infants and their physical assessment. The situation could have been extended to present a fuller picture of what nurses can do in such a setting, and a more complete coverage of the infant's and mother's needs in the situation. The simulation could then have been developed further to include having the infant seen in a pediatric clinic because of, for example, hypothyroidism, congenital dysplasia of the hip, or the like. Please note that the exercise is not complete but could constitute the beginning of a written simulation designed to assess a student's functioning in a mock Well Child Clinic.

Instructions for Taking the Test: There are several sections to this exercise with a list of choices for each section. For some sections, you are to choose only one option, while for other sections you are directed to choose as many as you think are indicated. Each section is prefaced by a specific directive telling you whether to choose only one or more than one. Since sections are not necessarily given in the order you would use them, it is essential that you follow the directions explicitly as they are revealed in the answer spaces. *(These answer sheets are not treated with the special material that would make the answers invisible until they are purposely revealed. Therefore, the answers are listed separately at the end of the exercise. If the latent image were used for the answer sheets, appropriate instructions for their use would need to be included.)†*

In taking this test, be sure to do each of the following:
1. Read the opening scene.
2. Start with Section A, make your first choice, and check the information given in the answer section. The end of the answer is indicated by an asterisk*.
3. Continue with Section B and follow the instructions given next to your choice(s).
4. Continue with the exercise until you are given the information that the problem is terminated.

   You will have 30 minutes to complete this exercise. *(This particular time limit is arbitrary.)*

   The exercise will be scored on a 3-point scale:

Essential to do	=	+1
Neutral	=	0
Essential to avoid	=	−1

(The scoring selected for this exercise is also arbitrary, since no panel of experts has reviewed the exercise and reached consensus on what constitutes appropriate action for each option.)

Client Situation I

Opening Scene
Mrs. Marie Gabriel, 22 years old, brings her 6-week-old daughter, Susie, to the Well Child Clinic for her first visit. Susie is the Gabriels' only child. Mrs. Gabriel tells you that Susie is a "good baby and rarely cries."

Continue with Section A
SECTION A
You would now (Choose
ONLY ONE):
1. Ask Mrs. Gabriel for   1.
   clarification of her
   comment
2. Assess Susie's physical   2.
   abilities
3. Take Susie's weight   3.
   and height
4. Assure Mrs. Gabriel   4.

---

†The material that appears in italics is not part of the test. It has been included as further, more specific, information on the test.

that young infants
are usually good
5. Question Mrs. Gabriel   5.
about Susie's devel-
opment since birth
6. Check Susie's vital   6.
signs

SECTION B
You would now (Select
AS MANY as you wish):
7. Do a physical assess-   7.
ment of Susie if you
have not already done
so
8. Teach Mrs. Gabriel the   8.
essentials of growth
and development of
young infants
9. Obtain a history of   9.
Susie's growth and
development if you
have not already done
so
10. Ask Mrs. Gabriel how   10.
Susie is eating her
cereal
11. Acquaint Mrs. Gabriel   11.
with the need for
Susie to start her
immunizations at this
visit
12. Orient Mrs. Gabriel to   12.
the clinic routines

SECTION C
In performing the physical
assessment of Susie, you
include testing of the
following reflexes. (Select
AS MANY of those
reflexes as are normally
present in infants of
Susie's age):
13. Landau reflex   13.
14. Moro reflex   14.
15. Parachute reflex   15.
16. Rooting reflex   16.
17. Sucking reflex   17.
18. Tonic neck reflex   18.

SECTION D
Continuing with the
assessment of Susie's
physical status, you are
particularly interested in
(Select AS MANY as

you consider particularly
important):

19. Hearing	19.
20. Vision	20.
21. Appearance of eyes	21.
22. Appearance of skin	22.
23. Anterior fontanel	23.
24. Posterior fontanel	24.
25. Umbilical area	25.
26. Position of feet	26.
27. Symmetry of gluteal folds	27.

SECTION E

In obtaining a history of
Susie's growth and devel-
opment from Mrs. Gabriel,
you are especially
interested in gathering
data relative to (Select
AS MANY as you consider
especially important):

28. Pattern of elimination	28.
29. Dietary pattern	29.
30. Sleep pattern	30.
31. Socialization	31.
32. Birth weight	32.
33. Tooth eruption	33.
34. Eye-hand coordina- tion	34.
35. Ability to sit with or without support	35.

. . . et cetera

Client Situation I: Some Suggested Answers

SECTION A
1. She says that she thought all babies cried a lot but Susie doesn't except when she's wet or hungry*
2. All fall within the normal range*
3. Weight 10 lb. 6 oz. (4.8 kg.), Height 22 in. (56 cm.)*
4. Done*
5. She says that to her knowledge, it's been normal*
6. Temperature 98.4 F. (36.8 C.), Pulse 130, Respirations 36*

SECTION B
7. Turn to Section C*
8. Done*
9. Turn to Section E*
10. Mrs. Gabriel tells you she hasn't started to give Susie cereal as yet*
11. Mrs. Gabriel says she thought it was not begun until 2 months of age*
12. Done*

SECTION C

13. Not present. Turn to Section D*
14. Present.   Turn to Section D*
15. Not present. Turn to Section D*
16. Present.   Turn to Section D*
17. Present.   Turn to Section D*
18. Present.   Turn to Section D*

SECTION D

19. Turns head toward side from which mother's voice is coming*
20. Is able to follow bright objects from side to side*
21. Strabismus present*
22. Mongolion spots present*
23. Open*
24. Closed*
25. No redness, moisture, or odor*
26. No clubbing present*
27. Asymmetrical—one higher than the other*

SECTION E

28. Has two soft bowel movements a day and voids "a lot"*
29. Takes 5 or 6 ounces of Similac five times a day and takes a long time to eat; gets no solids*
30. Falls asleep during or right after a bottle and sleeps between 18 and 20 hours a day*
31. Responds to mother's voice by smiling and waving arms and kicking legs*
32. 8 lb. 3 oz. (3.8 kg.)*
33. None*
34. Poorly developed*
35. Unable to sit with or without support*

. . . End of exercise

133

REFERENCES

1. Andrew, B. J.   An approach to the construction of simulated exercises in clinical problem-solving. *J. Med. Educ.* 47:952, 1972.
2. Barro, A. R.   Survey and evaluation of approaches to physician performance measurement. *J. Med. Educ.* 48:1048, 1973.
3. Barrows, H. S., and Abrahamson, S.   The programmed patient: A technique for appraising student performance in clinical neurology. *J. Med. Educ.* 39:802–805, 1964.
4. Barrows, H. S.   *The Programmed Patient: Evaluation and Instructions in Clinical Neurology.* In J. P. Lysaught and H. Jason (Eds.), *Self-Instruction in Medical Education*—Proceedings of Second Rochester Conference. Rochester, N.Y.: The Rochester Clearing House, University of Rochester, 1965.
5. Barrows, H. S.   Simulated patients in medical teaching. *Can. Med. Assoc. J.* 98:674–676, 1968.
6. Barrows, H. S.   *Simulated Patients (Programmed Patients).* Springfield, Ill.: Charles C Thomas, 1971.
7. Bashook, P. G.   A conceptual framework for measuring clinical problem-solving. *J. Med. Educ.* 51:109, 1976.
8. Berner, E. S., Hamilton, L. A., Jr., and Best, W. R.   A new approach to evaluating problem-solving in medical students. *J. Med. Educ.* 49:666, 1974.
9. Bevis, E. O.   *Curriculum Building in Nursing: A Process.* St. Louis: C. V. Mosby, 1973.
10. Boyd, J. L., Jr., and Shimberg, B.   *Handbook of Performance Testing.* Princeton, N.J.: Educational Testing Service, 1971.
11. Center for Educational Development, University of Illinois College of Medicine.   *Check List for Crisis Situation #1; (2-year-old Male Swallowed Aspirin).* (Sponsored by Illinois State Medical Society and Illinois Regional Medical Program.) Presented at the Annual Meeting of the National Council of Measurement in Education, Chicago, 1972.
12. Center for Educational Development, University of Illinois College of Medicine.   *Problem in Patient Management, Patient TD. Self-Assessment for Continuing Education.* (Sponsored by Illinois State Medical Society and Illinois Regional Medical Program.) Presented at the Annual Meeting of the National Council of Measurement in Education, Chicago, 1972.
13. Clark, C. C.   Simulation gaming: A new teaching strategy in nursing education. *Nurs. Educator* 1:4, 9, 1976.
14. Consortium of Medical Schools to Test Applicants for Diagnostic and Patient Skills. *ETS Developments* 24:2, 1977.
15. Curtis, J., and Rothert, M.   An instructional simulation system offering practice in assessment of patient needs. *J. Nurs. Educ.* 11:23, 1972.
16. de Tornyay, R.   The effect of an experimental teaching strategy on problem-solving abilities of sophomore nursing students. *Nurs. Res.* 17:108, 1968.
17. de Tornyay, R.   Measuring problem-solving skills by means of the simulated clinical nursing problem test. *J. Nurs. Educ.* 7:3, 1968.
18. Dincher, J. R., and Stidger, S. L.   Evaluation of a written simulation format for clinical nursing judgment: A pilot study. *Nurs. Res.* 25:280, 281, 284, 1976.
19. Dowaliby, F. J., and Andrew, B. J.   Relationships between clinical competence ratings and examination performance. *J. Med. Educ.* 51:181, 1976.
20. Elstein, A. S., Kagan, N., and Shulman, L. S.   Methods and theory in the study of medical inquiry. *J. Med. Educ.* 47:85, 1972.

21. Fitzpatrick, R., and Morrison, E. J.   Performance and Product Evaluation. In R. L. Thorndike (Ed.), *Educational Measurement* (2nd ed.). Washington, D.C.: American Council on Education, 1971. Pp. 237–270.
22. Flagle, C. D.   The role of simulation in the health services. *Am. J. Public Health* 60:2386, 1970.
23. Frederiksen, N.   In-Basket Tests and Factors in Administrative Performance. In A. Anastasi (Ed.), *Testing Problems in Perspective.* Washington, D.C.: American Council on Education, 1966. Pp. 208–221.
24. Gezi, K., and Hadley, F.   Strategies for developing critical thinking. *J. Nurs. Educ.* 9:9, 1970.
25. Goran, M. J., Williamson, J., and Gonnella, J.   The validity of patient management problems. *J. Med. Educ.* 48:171, 176, 1973.
26. Gover, V. F.   The NPSI: A Nursing Performance Simulation Instrument. Paper presented at the Eighth American Nurses' Association Nursing Research Conference, Albuquerque, N.M., March 15–17, 1972. Pp. 12, 29.
27. Grier, M. R.   Decision making about patient care. *Nurs. Res.* 25:105, 1976.
28. Guetzkow, H. (Ed.).   *Simulation in Social Science.* Englewood Cliffs, N.J.: Prentice-Hall, 1962.
29. Hayman, J.   Games—a teaching strategy. *Nurs. Outlook* 25:302, 1977.
30. Henry George School of Social Sciences New York, N.Y. Brochure, Fall, 1977.
31. Hubbard, J. P.   Programmed Testing in the Examinations of the National Board of Medical Examiners. In *Proceedings of the 1963 Invitational Conference on Testing Problems.* Princeton, N.J.: Educational Testing Service, 1964, Pp. 49–63.
32. Hubbard, J. P.   An objective evaluation of clinical competence—new technics used by the National Board of Medical Examiners. *N. Engl. J. Med.* 272:1321, 1965.
33. Hubbard, J. P.   *Measuring Medical Education.* Philadelphia: Lea & Febiger, 1971. Pp. 43–44, 162–171.
34. Juul, D. H., Noe, M. J., and Nevenberg, R. L.   A Factor Analytic Study of Branching Patient Management Problems. Paper presented at the National Council on Measurement in Education, New York, 1977. Pp. 2, 7.
35. Lamont, C. T., and Hennen, B. K. E.   The use of simulated patients in a certification examination in family medicine. *J. Med. Educ.* 47:789, 791, 1972.
36. Lange, C. M.   Developing low-cost teaching materials. *Nurs. Outlook* 24:614, 1976.
37. Levine, H. G., and McGuire, C. H.   Role-playing as an evaluative technique. *J. Educ. Measure.* 5:1, 1968.
38. Levine, H. G., and McGuire, C. H.   The validity and reliability of oral examinations in assessing cognitive skills in medicine. *J. Educ. Measure.* 7:63, 1970.
39. McCarthy, W. H.   An assessment of the influence of cueing items in objective examinations. *J. Med. Educ.* 41:263, 266, 1966.
40. McGuire, C. H.   The oral examination as a measure of professional competence. *J. Med. Educ.* 41:267, 269–270, 1966.
41. McGuire, C. H.   A Proposed Model for the Evaluation of Teaching. In *The Evaluation of Teaching,* A Report of the Second Pi Lambda Theta Catena. Washington, D.C.: 1967. Pp. 85–108.
42. McGuire, C. H.   An Evaluation Model for Professional Education— Medical Education. In *Proceedings of the 1967 Invitational Conference on Testing Problems.* Princeton, N.J.: Educational Testing Service, 1968. Pp. 37–52.

43. McGuire, C. H., and Babbott, D. Simulation technique in the measurement of problem-solving skills. *J. Educ. Measure.* 4:1, 1967.
44. McGuire, C. H., Solomon, L. M., and Forman, P. M. (Eds.). *Clinical Simulations: Selected Problems in Patient Management* (2nd ed.). New York: Appleton-Century-Crofts, 1976.
45. McGuire, C. H., and Page, G. *The Assessment of Clinical Performance by Written and Oral Simulations. Report to the Faculty 1972-73.* Chicago: Center for Educational Development, University of Illinois College of Medicine, 1973.
46. McGuire, C. H., Solomon, L. M., and Bashook, P. G. *Construction and Use of Written Simulations.* New York: Psychological Corp., 1976.
47. McIntyre, H. M., McDonald, F., Bailey, J., and Claus, K. A simulated clinical nursing test. *Nurs. Res.* 21:429–432, 435, 1972.
48. National Board of Medical Examiners. *Annual Report 1976-77.* Philadelphia: National Board of Medical Examiners, 1977. Pp. 25, 26, 29.
49. Perry, L. C. The use of simulation with students having a community health nursing experience. *J. Nurs. Educ.* 12:20, 1973.
50. Peterson, C., Connelly, S., DePew, C., Cowden, M., and Mayer, G. *Teaching and Evaluating Synthesis in an Associate Degree Nursing Program—A Developmental Experience.* (League Exchange No. 107.) New York: National League for Nursing, 1975.
51. Rimoldi, H. J. A. The test of diagnostic skills. *J. Med. Educ.* 36:73, 1971.
52. Sumida, S. W. A computerized test for clinical decision making. *Nurs. Outlook* 20:458–460, 1972.
53. Thorndike, R. L. (Ed.) *Educational Measurement* (2nd ed.). Washington, D.C.: American Council on Education, 1971.
54. Twelker, P. A. A Basic Reference Shelf on Simulation and Gaming. In D. W. Zuckerman and R. E. Horn (Eds.), *The Guide to Simulation Games for Education and Training.* Cambridge, Mass.: Information Resources, 1970. Pp. 313–328.
55. Williamson, J. W. Assessing clinical judgment. *J. Med. Educ.* 40:180, 1965.

7. Simulated Clinical Laboratories

A nursing student arrives on the surgical unit and is assigned the preoperative care of a patient who is scheduled for a hysterectomy. The student has had the theory of that care in class and has practiced in the nursing skills laboratory at different times some of the aspects of care that comprise the preparation of a patient for surgery. But now the student has to put it all together and what's more, the instructor is going to evaluate her on the performance.

Is there something wrong in this situation? Very definitely yes! First, if the student has never had the opportunity to learn how and to practice putting it all together, it is unjustifiable to evaluate her at this time *unless* the purpose of the evaluation is to help the student to learn. That purpose is very different from the purpose of evaluating the student in order to determine a grade or to make a pass-fail decision. Second, could the student have practiced putting together several of the facets of preoperative care in a simulated laboratory and then have been evaluated on those aspects there before being confronted with a real patient, with all the intervening variables that exist in the real world of the hospital? While there is no guarantee that the student who does well in the simulated laboratory will do equally well in the real situation, neither is there a guarantee that practicing in the real world will ensure competence in that world. Practicing in the simulated laboratory spares real patients unnecessary exploitation and, if you will, experimentation. In the simulated laboratory, the student is free to experiment within the parameters of the laboratory facilities *and* under the instructors' watchful eyes.

As can be determined from the literature and in casual discussions with faculty members, many and perhaps most schools of nursing have a student learning or nursing skills laboratory that contains equipment necessary for patient care as well as a variety of audiovisual and written materials. How these facilities are used apparently varies greatly. Some laboratories may be staffed by junior faculty members, some staffed by regular faculty members who rotate the responsibility for supervision among them, some by ancillary or nonhealth-related personnel, and, lastly unmanned at all. The hours of availability apparently are variable, too, from open access around the clock, weekends included, to very limited periods, with some of the restrictions being imposed by school or university decree. While I support the concept of peer learning, in the absence of an instructor, there are times when it is more like the blind leading the blind. If the student is alone in the learning laboratory and has questions that cannot be answered by the available materials, what does she do? Or what if the student perpetuates the same mistakes over and over again? I advocate the use of instructors in the nursing skills laboratory and there should be ready access to those laboratories, not necessarily 24 hours a day, but more than the conventional 7- or 8-hour day, 5 days a week, if we are to meet the needs of students as we purport to do.

WHEN SIMULATED LABORATORIES SHOULD
BE USED AND WHY

Because the "when" and the "why" are so interrelated, it is hard to separate the two and they therefore shall be discussed together. Simulated
laboratories should be used when it is more economical in terms of access
(is the hospital or clinical facility located at some distance to the school?),
when several students can be accommodated rather than providing experience for one, when equipment can be reused (e.g., repackaging a "sterile"
set), or when the equipment or materials is expensive. And there are times
when it is just more feasible to use a mock laboratory. Certainly the simulated laboratory should be used when it is safer to do so, both for the
student and the patient. I specifically mean when it is safer *not* to practice
on a real patient. In the mock laboratory the student is free to adapt care,
alter intervention and ministrations, and what is crucial, to make mistakes.

There are times when it would be desirable to use a simulated laboratory
to condense time. In the real world, elapsed time may prevent many students from getting a complete picture of a particular situation. A simple
example would be being with a patient from the first stage of labor through
the first hour postpartum. How many students have the opportunity to
stay with a woman throughout the labor and delivery cycle? In a laboratory (as in a patient-centered paper-and-pencil test), a programmed patient
could be directed to go rapidly from one stage to the next with the elapsed
time being a matter of minutes as compared to the hours of a typical and
real labor and delivery. Of course, in the not too distant future, computers
and computer-controlled manikins (a highly sophisticated Mrs. Chase) will
make such practices easier and more feasible. However, for the present
we must be content with utilizing the simulated laboratory to its maximum, allowing students to handle equipment, manipulate it, practice with
it, and feel comfortable using it before being required to perform those
skills on or with a real patient.

HOW SIMULATED LABORATORIES CAN
BE USED IN EVALUATION

In addition to their use in teaching—the most common one—simulated
laboratories can be very useful for evaluation. The simplest way to use a
simulated laboratory for this purpose is to assess each student's ability to
perform each of the procedures that are required for patient care. There
should be a checklist of some kind by which the evaluator can systematically check off each of the steps or elements that comprise the procedure. Evaluator time should not be spent in unnecessary writing or in
observing activities unrelated directly to the task.

Another method is to evaluate all of the students on each of the procedures deemed essential by the faculty while the other procedures can be
evaluated in the clinical situation when they occur. (This assumes that the
student would have been allowed time to learn the procedure before being
evaluated.)

Still another method is to assign students at random to one or more of the procedures under the assumption that if the student performs satisfactorily on that one (or more) procedure, she is likely to perform satisfactorily on the others. This method is not as satisfactory as the other two because it may be a lucky or unlucky sample for that student. It would be better to have as many samples of the student's behavior as possible. No pass-fail decision should be made on the basis of only one such observation of performance.

Another method more closely resembles actual patient care and is therefore likely to be better accepted by the students. They hopefully will identify more quickly with this method since it should appear more relevant. It involves the design of a patient situation using a variety of materials and evaluation methods. A patient's history is given only in enough detail to allow the student to decide what additional information is necessary before proceeding. The information could be written or it could be presented by a videotape or film. The student then performs an assessment. If it's a programmed patient, the information can be obtained verbally, or the student could select the information from among a list of data, as in a written simulation. When the nursing care plan has been written, the student could then be asked to order the priorities and carry out one or more of the identified measures in a simulated fashion. Obviously the scoring of such an examination will not be as readily accomplished as would a paper-and-pencil test, but the information gained from this method of assessment is likely to be worth the effort. The key to the scoring is the identification of critical elements that students must perform safely and a set of criteria for each of the procedures, against which each student will be compared—criterion-referenced, not norm-referenced. Faculty agreement as to the critical components of care is essential, regardless of the method employed. When a student has satisfactorily performed a procedure, then all faculty will know what that "satisfactory" signifies.

HOW SIMULATED LABORATORIES HAVE BEEN USED

What follows is a review of the literature, and although an attempt was made to find all relevant references in the fields of medicine and nursing, it is conceivable that a number of important ones have been overlooked. Article titles and abstracts, when available, do not always include the fact that simulation was involved. First to be discussed are those references from the field of medicine and second, those from nursing, generally starting with simulation laboratories in use for teaching purposes, followed by their application to evaluation.

A highly sophisticated (and very expensive) simulator was developed for use in training physicians to perform endotracheal intubations [1, p. 515]. Sim One, the computer-controlled manikin who looks life-like, was able to simulate certain human behaviors such as breathing, blinking the eyes, opening and closing the mouth, responding to the administration of drugs, and dying. In addition, the heart beat and pulse rates were synchronized. Since the manikin was computer-linked, the responses occurred "automatically" as a result of physician intervention. The physician performed the endotracheal intubation on Sim One in the same way it would have been performed in the operating room. Since the manikin's responses were in real time, Sim One's eyes would close and unconsciousness would occur in a matter of seconds following the administration of the anesthetic drug.

As can readily be seen, the use of the manikin for learning a potentially hazardous procedure was especially advantageous. Countless patients were thereby saved from the possibility of developing complications such as tracheal edema as a result of trauma suffered during the intubation.

Evaluation of the physician's proficiency was not done by direct observation nor was there any indication of objectives having been developed. Rather, an audit of appropriate patients' charts was carried out by members of the Department of Anesthesiology, who were asked to rate the physician's performance as either acceptable or unacceptable on the basis of the data contained in the charts. Results of the use of the simulator showed that physicians reached proficiency levels in a shorter time period than did those trained without the use of Sim One. Thus the use of the simulator also saved time as well as "posing significantly less threat to patient safety [1, p. 519]."

Sim One could be a milestone for both teaching and evaluation. Since the computer software was probably the most expensive part of the development of the simulator, we can benefit from what has been done and build on that model, and at considerably less expense. Other manikins of both sexes and of various ages could be developed for use in both teaching and evaluation. An example that comes to mind is a Sim One Junior—a 4-year-old who screams and carries on when approached with his intramuscular injection, and when the attempt is made to give him the injection, seems to be greased as if ready to swim the English Channel. Or, a normal primigravida in labor who has contractions that can be monitored by the nurse, or one who is in the transition phase and shouts at the nurse, "Leave me alone—get out of here!" or one who is expecting twins. At this time, there are still many hospitals that do not have monitoring equipment so nurses do need to know how to time contractions and obtain fetal heart rates. In addition to learning how to carry out these nursing measures, the simulators can be used for the purpose of evaluation. An ever-increasing cry over the dearth of experiences for students in the care of maternity patients could be partially alleviated by the provision of such a Mrs. Sim.

I have neither heard nor read about any further developments or use, or both, of Sim One but perhaps the methodology will not be lost. Hopefully, some creative faculty members, given some funding, will pursue this innovative approach to teaching and evaluation that offers so many advantages, only some of which are presently recognized.

Three simulation devices in ophthalmology and one in cardiology were used to teach some of the skills needed by physicians in a physical diagnosis course [17]. The models enabled medical students to identify pathologies of the eye, to examine the fundus systematically, "to develop skills in screening patients for strabismus [17, p. 443] ," and "to practice identification of heart sounds, rhythms, and murmurs [17, p. 444] ." The authors discuss the use of an objective test specifically designed to evaluate the students' ability to perform "the skills specified for each one of the four simulators [17, p. 444] ." The skills included such behaviors as "localize hemorrhage according to quadrant" and "recognize normal versus abnormal disc [17, p. 444] ." Since the skills are stated in behavioral terms, one wonders if, in fact, the test was a performance test rather than an objective test. Because of the success of the simulation tools for their intended purpose in this situation, other models have been investigated. When I visited the laboratory in 1972, they did have additional simulators, one of which was a gynecological model.

One variation of a simulated laboratory involves the use of "programmed" patients in a mock-up of a physician's office [14]. The simulated patients were played by actors from a local theatrical group in the manner described by Barrows [2]. The purpose of this examination for physicians in the practice of family medicine was certification and included evaluating the physician's ability to interact with patients and having him demonstrate his attitudinal skills. The scoring system is described and involves the weighting of the skills according to the opinions of the members of the examination committee. The procedure used for conducting the examination is also described, an important consideration when one is aiming to standardize, to the degree possible, the conditions of administration of an examination. Also discussed are Hermann's [11] criteria for assessing the validity of simulations. Finally, scores attained on the simulated test are correlated with those obtained on the other parts of the examination.

Over the years nursing service administrators have complained about the lack of proficiency in basic nursing skills—the how-to-do—of many graduates of baccalaureate degree nursing programs. Undoubtedly there are many factors that contribute to this deficit, not the least of which is the lack of opportunity to practice those nursing skills. "Teach them the principles of nursing practice, the theory underlying performance, and they'll be able to meet the physical needs of patients," is typical of the comments of faculty members in those schools turning out graduates ill-prepared to practice. Of course such an assumption by those faculty members is not justifiable on any grounds! That the problem exists is documented by Goldsberry [9, p. 46], among others, who describes the experiences of staff in a community health agency. Among the deficits noted, one was "in baseline facility in technical procedures [9, p. 47] ." She goes on to describe the orientation program designed to improve the competencies of those nurses.

A description of a simulated laboratory in a baccalaureate degree nursing program, the self-instructional materials that were used in the laboratory, and the staffing pattern in the laboratory are all included in the article "A Model for a Nursing Media Center" [12]. Five registered nurse instructors were available whenever the laboratory was open, and they assisted the nursing students in whatever way they could, including occasional testing, although no additional information is given about the nature of the testing. A picture of a portion of the college laboratory shows video screens at each bedside as well as some of the other equipment available to students. Since the purpose of the article was not to describe the evaluation methodology used in the laboratory, one would hope that nursing faculty would have followed up the description of the laboratory with the effects of its use, students' reactions to it, and the results obtained since its inception.

The use of an anesthetized dog whose chest has been opened is an effective method for teaching nurses cardiovascular physiology [8, p. 302]. An important aim of this program is to relate the effects of the students' actions to the nursing care of patients. Although not universally applicable to simulated nursing laboratories, this method demonstrates how creative simulated laboratories can be. The authors include the activities of the nurse-trainees during the experiment, the physiological observations they were to make, and the relevance of the activities and observations to nursing. How and whether the nurse-trainees were evaluated on completion of the experiment is not discussed, but the points listed in the column "Relevance to Nursing" [8, pp. 306–308] could easily have been the basis for the development of objective test questions. The development of a laboratory examination based on this specific content would not be quite so easy, however.

The analysis of a nursing procedure, a bed bath, was used as the basis for a discussion about the teaching and learning of psychomotor skills [10]. According to the author, "A factor analysis familiar to nurses is the 'procedure' in which the task is broken down into its component parts." While I would agree that it is necessary to make each behavior discrete in order to evaluate by direct observation the ability of a nurse to carry out a procedure, I would not assign the label *factor analysis* to that method. Psychometric theory treats factor analysis in quite a different way, namely in a statistical way. An example of the way psychometricians define the term, in part, is "Any of several methods of analyzing the intercorrelations among a set of variables such as test scores [22]." Nevertheless, the identification of the terminal objectives—behavioral objectives in this case—of the bed bath procedure would be very useful in not only facilitating students' learning but in evaluating their ability to give a bed bath and in a college laboratory. The only requirement necessary in order to use the listed objectives in that procedure, assuming you agree with the objectives, is to put them in the form of a checklist and add the space for the material needed for identifying the student, the date, the instructor, and the like (see the checklist in Chap. 4). The same format would be equally appropriate for other nursing procedures that could be evaluated in a classroom or simulated laboratory.

A novel simulated nursing laboratory for use in teaching was described more than 10 years ago by Bitzer [3] and utilized a computer. The author notes that in the real clinical situation the student is unable to manipulate many of the variables "to see what happens" because of the need to maintain patient safety. However, in a simulated laboratory, feedback of patients' responses is possible [3].

Although not *directly* concerned with evaluation, Infante's book on the use of the clinical laboratory, *The Clinical Laboratory in Nursing Education* [13], contains much valuable information, some with special relevance to evaluation. Among the highlights are the following points. First, the clinical laboratory "should be used only when that goal cannot be accomplished in the classroom or college laboratory," and "should be utilized only when patients are necessary for the student to accomplish a learning objective [13, p. 23]." Secondly,

. . . adequate provision should be made for independent learning and practice in the multimedia laboratory and the simulated clinical laboratory. But then the student must be allowed the freedom to observe, plan, test, and evaluate his own activities in the clinical laboratory without the teacher hovering over him [13, p. 29].

Third,

The college laboratory, properly equipped as a simulated setting, provides the best opportunity for students to learn the parts. After the parts have been learned, the task in the clinical laboratory is to assimilate the parts [13, p. 35].

My justification for including so many of Dr. Infante's comments is that if the college laboratory were used more for evaluation when it is appropriate to do so, evaluation in the clinical laboratory would probably be more meaningful, more reliable, more valid (e.g., not evaluating communication skills when the nurse's ability to administer an enema is what should be evaluated), and less frustrating to students and faculty alike.

A criterion-referenced tool was developed to evaluate the ability of nursing students to give basic nursing care [26]. The example discussed by the authors involves catheterization, perhaps an irrelevant procedure since it is one used so infrequently. Following study of the procedure via a module in an autotutorial laboratory, the student is evaluated on that procedure in a simulated laboratory. The authors discuss the development of the tool from the writing of the objectives through the establishment of inter-rater reliability, although some aspects of the development are inadequately dealt with. Included in the discussion are: the decision to use a rating scale rather than a checklist, the scoring system employed, the revision of the tool based on the tryout and the subsequent inclusion of key (or critical) behaviors, and the criteria for judging satisfactory, minimally acceptable, or unsatisfactory performance.

The biggest criticism about this method is the apparent use of the tool in a cumulative way as opposed to a one-time observation of performance. For further discussion on this point, refer to the section on rating scales and checklists in Chapter 4. It would have been especially useful to have a sample of the tool depicted in the article. Many questions about the design and usefulness of the tool that the authors did not answer might have been taken care of, in part, by the tool itself.

A simulated clinical laboratory used for nursing students to learn and practice their skills was also used to evaluate their performance [7, p. 270]. Included in the practical examination were simulated clinical patient-care situations, student viewing of videotapes in order to evaluate the preoperative teaching a patient had received, and role-playing with a simulated patient. Movies, slides, and audiotapes were also used but how they were used is not discussed. What is an especially desirable practice in evaluation and not generally included is the development of an evaluation blueprint that the authors mention. It is one way that the decision can be made about how a particular point will be tested—is it a cognitive objective or a psychomotor one? The authors also pretested the items and developed criteria for satisfactory performance in each situation. Although patient-care situations were evaluated on an individual basis, other portions of the examination, for example, that based on the videotape, were administered to small groups of students. The authors also discuss the use of single-concept items, used for the most part early in the students' education, and multiple-concept items. They give an example of each type along with the criteria for judging successful attainment of each item.

Among the advantages of this type of examination cited by the authors, two deserve mention. First, the variables in a simulated setting can be controlled [7, p. 271], and second, the safety of real patients is not threatened. And if this type of simulated clinical laboratory examination were developed and used in a baccalaureate nursing program, we perhaps wouldn't hear so many complaints from students about unfair evaluation practices as they pertain to differences in the complexity of needs of patients they are assigned to for the purpose of evaluation.

Rines [20, p. 69], in a paper on evaluation, describes simulated work situations and includes role-playing, laboratory situations, mock delivery rooms, and mock medical aseptic units. She states that although these simulations cannot be precisely reproduced, they have the advantage of being safe and convenient, and "all the variables in the setting can be predicted, controlled and planned."

In addition, Rines discusses work samples, another kind of performance testing, and again credits Dr. Elizabeth Hagen as the reference. In these actual work situations, which she states should be administered under standardized conditions, process and product may be evaluated separately or jointly. Among the advantages listed are that such tests have greater face validity because they are realistic. A major disadvantage pertains to the inability to sample behaviors adequately.

In adapting what Rines has presented, I can see how some of the products and processes given in the work sample could be included in a simulated laboratory situation. The examples of dressing a wound, giving medications, and carrying out aseptic technique [20, p. 70] are certainly appropriate for adaptation in a simulated laboratory.

Peterson and colleagues [18] describe one nursing student's experience in a clinical testing situation designed to evaluate synthesis. After assessing that the needs of the assigned patient are being threatened, the student confers with her instructor and then proceeds to gather additional information before actually planning the patient's care. The student includes information about the patient's postoperative orders and then plans the care based on all of the information she has gathered. Again she confers with her instructor before implementing that care. Evaluation of the student's performance in administering nursing care is done by the instructor, who then discusses it with the student.

One reason I cited this particular reference in this chapter on simulated laboratories is that I can see modifications or adaptations, or both, of this model for clinical performance evaluation in a mock laboratory. If, for example, a patient could be presented—be it on film or videotape, or a programmed patient, or, though not as desirable, even a written description—up to the point of planning patient care, then all students could design the nursing care that that patient needs. Of course, an answer key would need to be prepared against which all students' plans would be compared.

Following the nursing care plan exercise, each of the students could be asked to demonstrate one of the identified measures, such as giving a bed bath, administering an injection, changing a dressing, or irrigating a nasogastric tube. A fair way to assign these procedures would be on a random basis. The availability of checklists for each of the procedures would greatly facilitate evaluation. As students progress in the program, more complex nursing care could be structured, with the student being asked to order priorities and carry out necessary measures according to those priorities. The above recommendation may not be an easily fulfilled one, but as others have said, a long walk begins with one step.

A college laboratory practical examination for associate degree nursing students is described by Simpson [21, p. 23]. Faculty in the college devised the examination in order to remedy some of the problems associated with direct observation of students' clinical performance in the real setting, in particular, those related to subjectivity and reliability. During the examination each of the stations in the college laboratory contained equipment and a typed card with the questions pertaining to that situation. As the students walked around the laboratory, they recorded the answers to the questions in the answer books they carried with them. The article contains samples of the items included in the examination. The questions are of the short answer fill-in type and are for the most part at a low cognitive level, that is, factual, recall, or recognition. Interestingly, the author assumes that if a student got a particular question right, the student knew more than the question asked. For example, a medication card is presented with the route of administration purposely omitted. The card contains the information that the codeine sulfate may be given every 4 hours (q. 4h.) p.r.n. Question 5 asks, "If this drug is given at 9 A.M., what would be the next earliest time that it could be given? _____[21, p.25]."
The author states, "In order to answer question 5, as well as to be able to

interpret what P.R.N. means and to apply the rule for administration of the drug under this order, the student must understand the pharmacology of codeine sulfate." Actually any knowledge of pharmacology of codeine sulfate, or any other drug for that matter, is not necessary in this instance. The question is simply asking what p.r.n. means, albeit in combination with q. 4h.

Another procedure tested in this examination involved reading a thermometer and identifying the type of thermometer it was. Granted that a student needs to be able to do this before progressing to more complex tasks, this procedure could be extended, perhaps at a later point in a student's education, to include the other vital signs.

The third procedure presented involved a catheter irrigation set and the principles of asepsis. Students were to decide which of two sets was sterile (set B had obviously been opened) and should be used for the irrigation, but then the students are told to open set B in order to identify equipment. It would be interesting to see the item analysis data on these items!

The amount of knowledge gained about a student's *cognitive* abilities in relation to the psychomotor skills was probably useful even with the level of questions presented. Of the 10 questions presented in the sample, nine are cognitive in scope and could have been presented in a typical paper-and-pencil test using diagrams or pictures. Only one question of those presented involves manipulative skills, which is unfortunate because the college laboratory practical examination could have been designed to test psychomotor skills. I am not advocating the elimination of testing the student's knowledge related to the procedural aspects of nursing care but rather that as much of the "doing" as possible be tested in the college laboratory. Although various procedures could be tested as separate entities (and probably should be, especially for beginning students), groupings of them might be designed as the student progresses in the program. Such groupings could be developed to simulate actual patient care. For example, as a student demonstrates readiness for more complex assignments, the student might be assigned (in the simulated laboratory) to the care of a toddler in a Croupette or mist tent. What are the nursing care activities that will be necessary in this situation? Let us say that because this child has an elevated temperature, his temperature will need to be checked more frequently than is the usual practice, and that he may need aspirin and a cool bath to reduce his temperature. The child's respiratory and pulse rates are also rapid so that these too will need to be monitored. In addition, oral fluids are to be encouraged, fluid intake and urinary output are to be recorded, and an antibiotic is to be administered every 6 hours. This patient situation is a relatively common one, especially in the northeast region of this country in the middle of winter. Now how much of this, the "putting it together," could be tested in a simulated clinical laboratory practical examination?

Another "walk around" examination in a simulated laboratory in use in an associate degree nursing program is described by Petrovich [19]. This kind of examination is used in two nursing courses and requires "the student to observe and to demonstrate manual dexterity related to skills that the student should have mastered by the time of the exam." What is being planned is that students will have their performance of technical skills videotaped and when satisfied with their own performance, will turn it in for the instructor to evaluate. The author states, "This method gets not only at the technical skill, but at self-evaluation and judgment."

Use of a simulated clinical laboratory for testing some of the skills of nursing students in a community college is described by Eveslage [6]. In a matter of less than a page of text, she discusses the procedure, including the set-up and scoring methodology. Performance criteria guidelines are used by the instructors. She says, "Instructors feel that the extra time, money, and energy spent on simulation for evaluation are well worthwhile." One's curiosity is aroused about further developments by this faculty!

A graduate of the Associate in Applied Sciences external degree program in New York has written an interesting account of her experience in the program [25]. What is most important to the topic under discussion in that article is her expression of the worth of the clinical performance examination in terms of certifying competence.

It both identifies and tests the behaviors that can be expected of its graduates upon employment. It does so through the critical elements of care that are specified and must be successfully demonstrated by the student for each area of nursing care [25, p. 431].

This viewpoint expresses my feelings about what faculties should now be doing with and for their students before they graduate: certifying the clinical competence of those students. If evaluation of skills were done more objectively, more comprehensively, and more reliably, whether in the simulated laboratory or in the real clinical situation, or a combination of both, graduates would probably feel more confident about their skills and certainly employers would be happier with their new employees.

The most comprehensive and highly developed documented simulated laboratory examination in nursing is that of the New York State Regents External Degree Program. The simulation phase of the examination (the other part of the clinical performance examination involves actual patient care) includes the application of a sterile dressing and the preparation and administration of oral, intramuscular, and intravenous medications. Candidates must have 100 percent accuracy in carrying out the critical elements specified for each procedure.

If one is unfamiliar with the development, content, and execution of this simulated laboratory examination or the actual patient care performance examination, several references by Dr. Lenburg will be informative [15, 16]. Available from the University of the State of New York Regents External Degree Programs are two other extremely useful documents [5, 23]. Before one embarks on the development of a simulated laboratory test, I advise studying these four references.

AN EXAMPLE OF A SIMULATED
LABORATORY EXAMINATION

What follows is an example of a test that could be administered in a mock laboratory. It was designed to be used in a course dealing with pediatric nursing content. Although much of the examination involves knowledge in the cognitive domain, some of it does pertain to psychomotor skills. The inclusion of such content will mollify those critics who contend that psychomotor skills should not be tested in the absence of cognition about those skills.

A scoring system has not been constructed because the examination is not complete. In addition, faculties may prefer other answers and make substitutions. It would be essential for faculty deciding to employ such an examination to agree on both the content and the acceptable answers. I would suggest using a book such as Wood's [24] for designing the checklists for the procedural sections of the examination.

A Sample Simulated Laboratory Examination

Instructions: Read the patient situation and think about the implications for nursing care in that situation. Then proceed to the questions, answering them as concisely but as completely as possible. For those that require a written response, use your examination book. Credit will *not* be given for length of answers but for the content.

Patient Situation

At 3 A.M., Johnny Nero, 18 months old, is admitted to the pediatric unit with a diagnosis of acute laryngotracheobronchitis and acute bilateral otitis media. His temperature on admission is 103.4°F (39.7°C), his respiratory rate is 42 per minute, and his apical heart rate is 132 per minute. Arterial blood gases have been drawn. Johnny's mother is with him.

The doctor's orders for Johnny include the following:

Croupette with oxygen at 10 L/min.

Tempra 0.6 ml. p.o. and q.4h. thereafter for temperature higher than 101°F (38.3°C)

500 ml. 2½ percent dextrose in normal saline intravenously to run for 12 hours.

Ampicillin 300 mg. q.4h. X 6 doses, IV. (If IV is discontinued after 24 hours, ampicillin will be given orally. Call doctor for new orders.)

Clear fluids by mouth ad lib.

Call doctor if respiratory distress increases.

1. On admission, what information should most certainly be obtained from Johnny's mother?

2. What information should be obtained from Mrs. Nero but at a later time?

3. Which of the doctor's orders should be carried out first?

   Why?

   Second?

   Why?

   Third?

   Why?

4. Write a nursing care plan for Johnny as it should appear in the Kardex.

5. Select one of the first four procedures and carry it out to the extent possible from beginning to end.

6. At the discretion of the instructor, questions such as the following may be asked of you after completion of the procedure.

   A. Croupette with oxygen
      1. What is the advantage of the fine mist?

2. Why is the oxygen administered at 10 liters per minute rather than at 5 liters per minute as it might be by mask?
3. Why must the bottom of the plastic canopy be tucked in?
4. What measures should be instituted to promote Johnny's comfort and to prevent chilling?

B. Tempra administration
1. What would you say to Johnny before giving him the Tempra?
2. Why is it best to give the medication by dropper rather than mixed with a quantity of milk or juice?

C. Intravenous fluids
1. What are the signs of infiltration?
2. Which manifestations would be most indicative of overly rapid administration of intravenous fluids?
3. Why are oral fluids administered as well as intravenous fluids?

D. Ampicillin administration
1. Can the medication be prepared ahead of time?
2. What is the most common untoward effect of ampicillin?

SOME SUGGESTED ANSWERS FOR THE SIMULATED LABORATORY EXAMINATION

1. A. How did she attempt to help Johnny at home and did she give him any medication?
   B. Does she have any other children? Is someone with them? Can the nurse assist her in making plans for their care while Johnny is in the hospital?
   C. Has Johnny ever received penicillin before? Does he have any allergies?
   D. Does she understand what is happening to Johnny?
   E. How does Johnny drink fluids—from a bottle, glass, or cup?

2. A. Does she have a regular place to go for health care for her child(ren)?
   B. How does she manage at home when her child(ren) is/are sick?
   C. Does she know how to manage fever and vomiting and other manifestations of illness in children?
   D. What is the home environment like, e.g., heat, humidity, etc.?

3. *First.* The Croupette.
   Why. It facilitates respiratory exchange and relieves dyspnea, therefore easing the child's anxiety.
   Second. Fluid administration.
   Why. To correct dehydration, reduce fever, provide vehicle for administration of medication, and liquify respiratory secretions.
   Third. Administer the medications.
   Why. The sooner they are administered, the sooner the therapeutic effect will be achieved. Deterioration of the child's condition is also likely to be prevented.

4. Nursing Care Plan

Problem	Nursing Action	Rationale
Respiratory difficulty on inspiration	1. Place infant in Croupette	1. Humidified air will liquify secretions
	2. Regulate O_2 at 10L/min.	2. Overoxygenation will further depress respiration
	3. Elevate head on pillow	3. Relieves upward pressure on diaphragm
	4. Observe every 15 min. for signs of increasing hypoxia: a. Restlessness b. Inspiratory retraction c. Pallor progressing to cyanosis d. Sweating e. Increasing pulse and respiratory rates	4. If intubation or tracheostomy should become necessary, it should be performed before the infant becomes completely exhausted
Fear of the hospital setting	1. Place a chair by the bed for his mother	1. He will probably become frightened if he cannot see his mother
	2. Give him a familiar object from home to hold	2. Toddlers often feel more secure with familiar objects
	3. Approach him carefully and gently	3. Forceful approach by a stranger may frighten him
Discomfort has led to decreased fluid intake	1. Provide his mother with clear fluid according to child's preference and encourage her to offer him frequent small sips	1. Infant will probably accept fluids best from his mother. Small sips will help prevent vomiting. If oral intake is adequate, IV may be discontinued
	2. If mother seems fatigued, nurse should offer fluids to the child. Don't force them	2. Forced fluids will increase anxiety and aggravate respiratory distress
	3. Secure IV with arm board. Regulate at 42 mini-drops per minute	3. Integrity of IV must be maintained. Fluids must be regulated to prevent over- or underhydration

Problem	Nursing Action	Rationale
Elevated temperature	1. Administer oral Tempra slowly with dropper. Mother may do this if she has done it satisfactorily at home	1. Antipyretic. Child will probably take it better from mother
	2. Retake rectal temperature in 30 minutes unless infant is sleeping. If infant is asleep wait 45 minutes to 1 hour	2. It is important to prevent further temperature elevation, but child also needs rest
	3. Offer fluids as outlined above	3. Adequate hydration can help reduce fever
Rubbing ears and seems to have ear pain.	1. Administer IV ampicillin as soon as possible	1. Prompt reduction of infection will lessen pain
	2. Administration of Tempra every four hours as needed	2. Tempra also has analgesic properties

5. *(Each of the procedures should have a checklist that is used to evaluate the student's performance. Essential elements should be identified and criteria for determining either pass or fail should be stated.*)*

6. A. Croupette with oxygen.
   1. The smaller size droplets are inhaled deeper to moisten and liquify secretions thereby increasing effectiveness of treatment.
   2. The oxygen is dispersed into a larger area, requiring a higher liter flow to achieve desired oxygen concentration.
   3. Oxygen is heavier than air and will escape unless the exits are closed.
   4. Johnny's gown or pajamas and bed clothing should be changed as often as necessary to keep him dry.

   B. Tempra administration
   1. "Johnny, here is your medicine. Open your mouth."
   2. If the medication is mixed with a large amount of fluid, the child might not take it all and it would be impossible to tell how much of the medication he actually received. Also, it is unwise to mix medications with food. It may affect the child's future intake of that food.

   C. Intravenous fluids
   1. Swelling around the site of needle insertion and hardness of the area.
   2. Increase in the rate of respiration, shallow respirations, grunting respirations, and possibly the use of the accessory muscles of respiration.
   3. Oral fluids will provide the child with additional fluids since

*The material that appears in italics is not part of the test. It has been included as further, more specific, information on the test.

the amount ordered intravenously is not enough to meet the child's daily needs. In addition it is a normal activity with which the child is familiar in an unfamiliar stressful situation.

D. Ampicillin administration
   1. Yes, but only up to one hour beforehand. On the other hand, the oral suspension when reconstituted is stable, if refrigerated, for up to 14 days.
   2. Hypersensitivity reactions are most common and include urticaria, dermatitis, rashes, and anaphylaxis.

REFERENCES

1. Abrahamson, S., Denson, J. S., and Wolf, R. M. Effectiveness of a simulator in training anesthesiology residents. *J. Med. Educ.* 44:515, 519, 1969.
2. Barrows, H. S. *Simulated Patients (Programmed Patients).* Springfield, Ill.: Charles C Thomas, 1971.
3. Bitzer, M. Clinical nursing instruction via the PLATO simulated laboratory. *Nurs. Res.* 15:144, 1966.
4. Boyd, J. L., Jr., and Shimberg, B. *Handbook of Performance Testing.* Princeton, N.J.: Educational Testing Service, 1971.
5. *College Proficiency Examinations—Regents External Degrees.* Albany, N.Y.: University of the State of New York, 1977.
6. Eveslage, M. M. Simulating clinical experience. *Nursing 76* 6:30, 1976.
7. Frejlach, G., and Corcoran, S. Measuring clinical performance. *Nurs. Outlook* 19:270, 271, 1971.
8. Fuller, E. D., and Dismukes, L. M. An open-chest preparation in the laboratory for teaching coronary care. *Nurs. Forum* 8:302, 306–308, 1969.
9. Goldsberry, J. From student to professional. *J. Nurs. Admin.* 7:46, 47, 1977.
10. Gudmundsen, A. Teaching psychomotor skills. *J. Nurs. Educ.* 14:23, 24, 1975.
11. Hermann, C. F. Validation problems in games and simulations with special reference to models of international politics. *Behav. Sci.* 12: 216, 1967.
12. Hoose, D. C. A model for a nursing media center. *Nurs. Outlook* 24:104, 105, 1976.
13. Infante, M. S. *The Clinical Laboratory in Nursing Education.* New York: John Wiley, 1975. Pp. 23, 29, 35.
14. Lamont, C. T., and Hennen, B. K. E. The use of simulated patients in a certification examination in family medicine. *J. Med. Educ.* 47:789, 1972.
15. Lenburg, C. B. *Criteria for Developing Clinical Performance Evaluation.* New York: National League for Nursing, 1976.
16. Lenburg, C. B. The external degree in nursing: The promise fulfilled. *Nurs. Outlook* 24:422, 1976.
17. Penta, F. B., and Kofman, S. The effectiveness of simulation devices in teaching selected skills of physical diagnosis. *J. Med. Educ.* 48:442–444, 1973.
18. Peterson, C., Connelly, S., DePew, C., Cowden, M., and Mayer, G. *Teaching and Evaluating Synthesis in an Associate Degree Nursing Program—A Developmental Experience.* League Exchange No. 107. New York: National League for Nursing, 1975. Pp. 67–69.
19. Petrovich, S. Evaluation Based on Philosophy and Objectives, Conceptual Framework, Curriculum Threads and Course Objectives. In National League for Nursing (Eds.), *Preparing the A.D. Graduate.* (Papers presented at a workshop by N.L.N. Council of A.D. Programs, Cincinnati, Ohio.) New York: National League for Nursing, 1977. P. 60.
20. Rines, A. R. The Process of Evaluation. In National League for Nursing (Eds.), *Preparing the A.D. Graduate.* (Papers presented at a workshop by N.L.N. Council of A.D. Programs, Cincinnati, Ohio.) New York: National League for Nursing, 1977. Pp. 69, 70.
21. Simpson, M. J. The "walk around" laboratory practical examination in evaluating clinical nursing skills. *J. Nurs. Educ.* 6:23, 25, 1967.

22. Stanley, J. C., and Hopkins, K. D. *Educational and Psychological Measurement and Evaluation.* Englewood Cliffs, N.J.: Prentice-Hall, 1972. P. 450.
23. Study Guide: Clinical Performance in Nursing Examination. Albany, N.Y.: The University of the State of New York, Regents External Degree Programs, 1975. (Mimeographed.)
24. Wood, L. A., and Rambo, B. J. (Eds.). *Nursing Skills for Allied Health Services* (2nd ed.). Philadelphia: W. B. Saunders, 1977.
25. Woodward, E. S. Reflections of an external degree graduate. *Nurs. Outlook* 24:429, 431, 1976.
26. Wyman, J., and Fernau, K. Developing a criterion-referenced tool. *Nurs. Outlook* 25:584, 1977.

Index